i

REBUILT RECOVERY

A JOURNEY WITH GOD

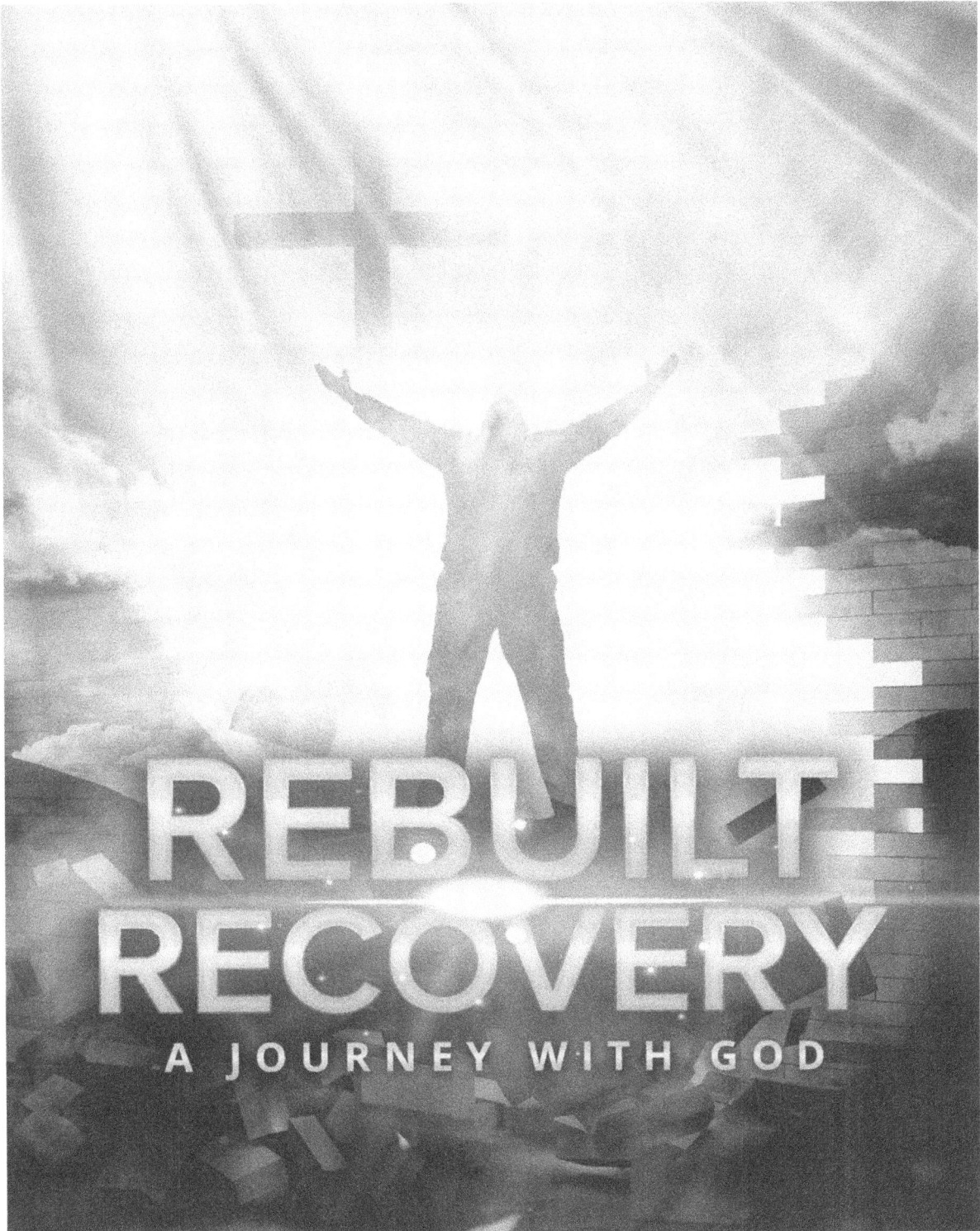

Glorious Hope Publishing

New Carlisle, Ohio

Rebuilt Recovery

A Journey with God

Book 2 – Knowing Yourself

By: Heather L. Phipps

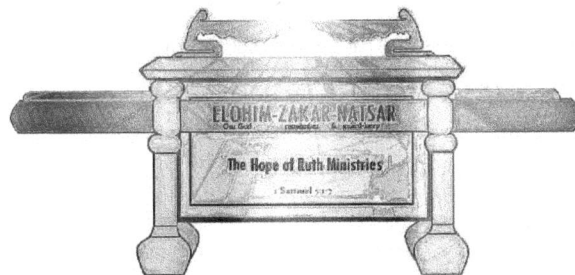

Rebuilt Recovery Is a Ministry of The Hope of Ruth Ministries Church

Glorious Hope Publishing

ISBN: 979-8-9852542-1-1 (Paperback)
Library of Congress Control Number: 2021922804

Glorious Hope Publishing
Hope of Ruth Ministries
307 Prentice Dr. New Carlisle, Ohio 45344
info@hopeofruthministries.com
www.hopeofruthministries.com

*Thank you to the following people
who gave their ideas, hearts,
and lives into making this book possible.*

Cindy Varghese

Summer Curtis

Alysha Allen

Justin Curtis

Annaka Schleinitz-Brooks

Jaycie Curtis

Camie Hawkins

Terri Allison

Contents

The Complete Rebuilt Series

Boxes and Symbols

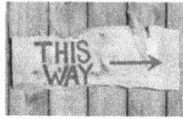

	These boxes have thoughts or questions involving your coach.

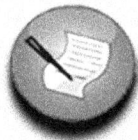

	These boxes contain additional tasks for your journey. Do not skip these tasks!

	These boxes contain tips with additional information to help understand or implement the topic being discussed.

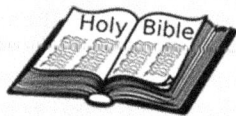

	This icon indicates scripture important to understanding the current topic.

	These boxes have important points for you to consider.

	"These boxes contain interesting quotes"

Disclaimer

The information contained in the *Rebuilt for Life* (online course), *Rebuilt Recovery*, or *Rebuilt Website* is for general information purposes only. The content is not intended to be a substitute for professional advice, diagnosis, or treatment, rather it is intended as a supplement to it. Always seek the advice of your mental health professional or other qualified health provider with any questions you may have regarding your condition. It is your responsibility to inform your mental health professional that you are using a *Rebuilt* service to aid your recovery. Never disregard professional advice or delay in seeking it because of something you have read or heard in *Rebuilt* materials, website, or courses.

Rebuilt coaches are not qualified counselors and do not take the place of certified professionals.

The information is provided by *The Hope of Ruth Ministries* and whilst we endeavor to keep the information up-to-date and correct, we make no representations or warranties of any kind, express or implied, about the completeness, accuracy, reliability, suitability, or availability with respect to the website, books, online course, the information, products, services, or related graphics contained on the internet or print materials for any purpose. Any reliance you place on such information is therefore strictly at your own risk.

In no event will we be liable for any loss or damage including without limitation, indirect or consequential injury, loss, or damage, or any injury, loss, or damage whatsoever arising from loss of life, relations, property, data, or profits arising out of, or in connection with, the use of the *Rebuilt* website, *Rebuilt for Life, Rebuilt Recovery,* or *Rebuilt Coaches.*

Every effort is made to keep the websites up and running smoothly. However, *The Hope of Ruth Ministries* nor *Rebuilt Recovery* takes no responsibility for, and will not be liable for, the coaches, website, software, or course being temporarily unavailable due to technical issues beyond our control.

COPYRIGHT NOTICE FOR SUPPLEMENTAL MATERIAL

EXTERNAL LINKS

Through the *Rebuilt* websites and courses, you may link to other websites, which are not under the control of *Rebuilt* or *The Hope of Ruth Ministries*. We have no control over the nature, content, and availability of such sites. The inclusion of any links does not necessarily imply a recommendation or endorse the views expressed within them.

Serenity Prayer

God, grant me the serenity
to accept the things I cannot change,
the courage to change the things I can,
and the wisdom to know the difference.

Living one day at a time,
enjoying one moment at a time;
accepting hardship as a pathway
to peace;

taking, as Jesus did,
this sinful world as it is,
not as I would have it;
trusting that You will make
all things right
if I surrender to Your will;

so that I may be reasonably happy
in this life
and supremely happy with You
forever in the next.

Amen.

Reinhold Niebuhr

Introduction to Book Two

Relationship with Self

Do you struggle constantly to believe in your ability or worth? Do you despise yourself when you lose control? Is anger a perpetual war in your heart? As life goes on, we often flip-flop between confidence and doubt. Can you imagine how freeing it might be to appreciate who you are and have confidence that you will respond well to life's challenges?

You are worthy of everything God has for you because He has made you worthy!

To have confidence in yourself, you need to know yourself. To have confidence in what God can or will do in you, you need to know who God says you are in Him. Know God. Know yourself.

Don't ask yourself if you are able, but if you believe God can make you able!

In This Book

Heart Check & Inventory
You will examine the condition of your heart using methods revealed in Scripture, and you will make an inventory of your life, revealing patterns that may expose the root of your problems.

Problematic Thinking & Stuck Points
You will learn how to identify the ideas keeping you stuck and to change patterns of problematic thinking.

Self-control
You will discover how to overcome overwhelming emotions.

Perseverance
You will learn to persevere when life seems beyond hope, even when you feel attacked from every direction.

Anger Management
You will discover strategies for controlling out-of-control anger and learn the difference between destructive and beneficial anger.

Anxiety & Fear Management
Fear manifests many ways. It is the greatest tool in the enemy's arsenal. You will learn to identify fear triggers and combat them.

Chapter Five

Heart Check & Inventory

Lesson 10 — Understanding What's Ahead

Before you begin Book Two, it's important to understand how this part of your journey will work. This is the meat of your journey—one of the most difficult and rewarding parts. This lesson explains each section of this book and the heart check exercise, which you will use throughout.

The Heart Check

The heart check helps you examine the current condition of your heart and reveals both the good and the bad things hidden within it. This helps you identify areas of denial or avoidance and brings them to light where you can deal with them. It is important to remember the purpose of the heart check is to discover problems, not fix them. **You must discover what is in your heart before change can happen!**

The Heart Check Plan

After completing all the heart checks in this book, you will review your answers to identify areas where you desire change. You will define the results you want to accomplish and set goals to achieve those results. At the end of this book, you will revisit your plan and evaluate both your progress and how your goals have changed since you began.

The Inventory

The inventory is an assessment of your life that examines your resentments, fears, and hurts, along with harm you may have caused others. The inventory worksheets will help expose patterns in your life that led to detrimental relationships and behaviors. You may continue to the lessons on coping skills while working on your inventory to help you progress. However, **do not continue to the next book until your inventory is complete.** Your coach has additional tools and activities to aid the inventory process.

Coping Skills

These lessons will help you identify and deal with obstacles you may encounter on your journey. Each lesson provides a tool or acrostic teaching about problematic thinking patterns, stuck points, perseverance, powerful emotions, and managing anger and anxiety. These coping skills will remain useful even after this journey.

> Do not continue without a coach. Now is a good time to find a strong accountability partner too—one who listens, keeps you balanced, and gives you support.

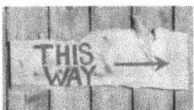

THIS WAY → This week, your coach will share an object lesson to illustrate the enemy's strongholds in your life and the changes that occur when you make God your only stronghold.

Heart Check

But the Lord said to Samuel, "Do not look on his appearance or on the height of his stature, because I have rejected him. For the Lord sees not as man sees man looks on the outward appearance, but the Lord looks on the heart." (1 Samuel 16:7)

The Lord sees the genuine condition of your heart. He knows your beginning, your end, and everything in between, yet His focus is never on the outside appearance. God does not worry about the job you have, the car you drive, or the size of your body. His first concern is the state of your heart.

Every way of a man is right in his own eyes, but the Lord weighs the heart. (Proverbs 21:2)

What Is the Heart?

When God speaks about the heart, He is referring to our core being: our mind, will, and emotions. The Lord examines our desires, our motives, our plans, our schemes, and how we understand people or situations.

We hide behind layers of walls, but the Lord looks at the person beneath the layers. God knows us better than we know ourselves. He knows our wrong thoughts and actions, even those **we cannot acknowledge in ourselves but are quick to see in others**. Only with the Lord can we recognize our true condition. We lack self-control when we do not understand why we do the things we do.

For I do not understand my own actions. For I do not do what I want, but I do the very thing I hate. (Romans 7:15)

For you say, I am rich, I have prospered, and I need nothing, not realizing that you are wretched, pitiable, poor, blind, and naked. (Revelation 3:17)

Ask the Lord to test your heart and reveal needed changes. He exposes things as we become open to seeing them.

Prove me, O Lord, and try me; test my heart and my mind. (Psalm 26:2)

Create in me a clean heart, O God, and renew a right spirit within me. (Psalm 51:10)

God's word helps us understand our heart. Scripture is a mirror which reflects the condition of our character.

For the word of God is living and active, sharper than any two-edged sword, piercing to the division of soul and of spirit, of joints and of marrow, and discerning the thoughts and intentions of the heart. (Hebrews 4:12)

Question to Ponder

10.1) Do you have questions or concerns before you continue?

Lesson 11 — The Tongue, Part 1

One way to test your heart is by checking what comes out of your mouth. Your words are an overflow of what is in your heart. There are hundreds of scriptures regarding our words.

The good person out of the good treasure of his heart produces good, and the evil person out of his evil treasure produces evil, for out of the abundance of the heart his mouth speaks. (Luke 6:45)

But what comes out of the mouth proceeds from the heart, and this defiles a person.
For out of the heart come evil thoughts, murder, adultery, sexual immorality, theft, false witness, slander. These are what defile a person. (Matthew 15:18 – 20)

It is not what goes into the mouth that defiles a person,
but what comes out of the mouth; this defiles a person. (Matthew 15:11)

Read James 3

James 3 is clear that no one is innocent regarding their tongue. It is the hardest member of the body to control. This chapter compares the tongue to a blazing forest, which can set the entire course of your life on fire. Like the rudder on a ship, your will drives your speech. A tongue "set on fire by hell" is an easy tool for the enemy to use—an untamable, restless evil full of deadly poison. Believers should never spew poison; they should only give life!

Below are several scriptures that deal with the power of our words. Read the reflections and then answer the questions that follow each Scripture.

The Lord hates a deceitful and divisive mouth
Scripture mentions seven things that are an abomination to the Lord. All seven are matters of the heart, and three involve the tongue: lies, false witness, and discord.

There are six things that the Lord hates, seven that are an abomination to him: haughty eyes, a lying tongue, and hands that shed innocent blood, a heart that devises wicked plans, feet that make haste to run to evil, a false witness who breathes out lies, and one who sows discord among brothers. (Proverbs 6:16 – 19)

Question to Ponder
11.1) How often have people's words hurt you? List as many times as you can remember.

Your words are your responsibility. You must guard your tongue. Each of us will give an account **for every idle word** we speak. God is serious about our words because unchecked words cause great harm; He equates them with death. Slander and lies ruin lives. Words can destroy one's spirit, reputation, and witness. Those whose words have hurt you **will** give an account to God, and you will give an account for careless and harmful words you speak.

I tell you, on the day of judgment people will give account for every careless word they speak, for by your words you will be justified, and by your words you will be condemned. (Matthew 12:36 – 37)

> ## Question to Ponder
> 11.2) How often have your words hurt others? List as many specific instances as you can remember.

Words have the power to cause death or produce life! Our words can encourage, pray, teach, correct, witness, counsel, bless others, and honor God.

Death and <u>life</u> are in the power of the tongue, and those who love it will eat its fruits. (Proverbs 18:21)

As Iron sharpens iron, one man sharpens another. (Proverbs 27:17)

> ## Question to Ponder
> 11.3) How often have your words benefited and brought life to others? List as many specific instances as you can remember.

Guard Your Words

Whoever guards his mouth preserves his life; he who opens wide his lips comes to ruin. (Proverbs 13:3)

How do you guard your tongue? We will not always say the right things, but we can limit the damage our tongue may cause. There is a popular saying, "We have two ears and one mouth so that we can listen twice as much as we speak." If we **are** listening, we **are not** speaking, and idle words cannot get us in trouble. Take this thought deeper. God also gave you two eyes to observe. Listening is not simply being quiet; it is seeing the meaning behind the speaker's words. Observe the speaker and ponder his words, and *your* words in response will be filled with wisdom and influence.

Listen
Listen to others before speaking and pay attention to instruction and correction.

Let every person be quick to hear, slow to speak, slow to anger. (James 1:19)

If one gives an answer before he hears, It is his folly and shame. (Proverbs. 18:13)

A fool takes no pleasure in understanding, but only in expressing his opinion. (Proverbs 18:2)

The ear that listens to life-giving reproof will dwell among the wise. (Proverbs 15:31)

The way of a fool is right in his own eyes, but a wise man listens to advice. (Proverbs 12:15)

Stop Talking

The best advice ever given: Only speak when you have something of value to say. Who gave that advice? God did. The more words you use, the more likely they will hurt someone. People place greater value on your words and message when you refrain from unnecessary speech.

Even a fool who keeps silent is considered wise; when he closes his lips, he is deemed intelligent. (Proverbs 17:28)

When words are many, sin is unavoidable, but he who restrains his lips is wise. (Proverbs 10:19)

Do you see a man who is hasty in his words? There is more hope for a fool than for him. (Proverbs 29:20)

Questions to Ponder

11.4) How well do you listen?

11.5) Do you consider the actual message someone is trying to convey, or do you seek ways to argue for your own perspective?

11.6) What changes could help you better guard your words? Commit to these changes.

Lesson 12 — The Tongue, Part 2

Gossip, Deception, and Lies, Oh My!

Has someone ever lied to you? It hurts, doesn't it? It is difficult to give trust to people capable of deceit. Lies don't just hurt our feelings; they destroy lives. People may mislead your thoughts or deceive you to act in ways you otherwise would not. They can take advantage of you, manipulate you, destroy your reputation, and involve you in legal disputes.

Deception takes many forms, from a blatant lie to subtle manipulation. It may present itself as a joke or a mistake. Deception disguised as kindness and flattery appeals to the ego while urging certain actions. Flattery is dangerous because it can manipulate you to act badly while feeling great.

Have you ever lied about your opinion of someone to protect his or her feelings? Your lie may lead others to have unreasonably high expectations, or it could cause them to feel shame and rejection. Pretending to be a friend while hiding your true feelings is deceptive and harmful.

Like a madman who throws firebrands, arrows, and death is the man who deceives his neighbor and says, 'I am only joking!' (Proverbs 26:18 – 19)

For such persons do not serve our Lord Christ, but their own appetites, and by smooth talk and flattery they deceive the hearts of the naive. (Romans 16:18)

The one who conceals hatred has lying lips, and whoever utters slander is a fool. (Proverbs 10:18)

His speech was smooth as butter, yet war was in his heart; his words were softer than oil, yet they were drawn swords. (Psalm 5521)

Keep your tongue from evil and your lips from speaking deceit. (Psalm 34:13)

> ### Questions to Ponder
>
> 12.1) Has anyone ever lied to you? How did their lies harm you?
>
> 12.2) Have you ever lied to anyone? What harm was caused to others by your lies? (Play this lie all the way out. Who may have been hurt beyond the person you lied to? What were the unintended consequences of your lie?)

Gossip and Malicious Words

Gossip is when lies or exaggerated truth are spoken **to** us or **about** us. It could be ridicule, sharing someone's personal information, or talking about a person's mistakes or flaws. In any situation, gossip unfairly influences other's opinions about an individual.

People frequently conceal gossip as concern or a prayer request. It may be hidden in a "warning" about someone. A person may justify gossip because the hearer of the gossip is aware of the situation. They may claim it is acceptable to discuss it because it is "common knowledge". However, **the further from the source information travels, the less truth is conveyed**. The truth is often contrary to an individual's perception of a situation.

No one wants another to share their business. It is the individual's choice to share information about their lives. The choice does not belong to another.

Gossip may not start with malicious intent. It may be genuine concern for someone, legitimate prayer needs, or a simple comment relating to another's experience. You may possess a genuine belief it was an acceptable topic to discuss. Get permission before sharing anything about an individual with another person.

> Every time you share anything <u>about someone who is not you</u>, your words have the potential to become twisted and misconstrued, and to spread.

You Are Responsible

What if you do not spread gossip, but surround yourself with people who do? Just as **you are accountable for your words** and those to whom you speak them, **you are also responsible for the gossip you hear.** Every word you let into your mind influences you. Listening to someone speak about another, whether it puts them in a positive or negative light, influences your opinion of them. Hearing a false understanding or perspective can turn you against a quality person, or toward believing a deceptive one. Gossip skews truth. You are not missing out if you refuse to listen to gossip.

An evildoer listens to wicked lips, and a liar gives ear to a mischievous tongue.
(Proverbs 17:4)

Questions to Ponder

12.3) What gossip and lies have harmed you?

12.4) When did you listen to gossip and with whom?

12.5) Have you ever spread gossip and lies to others?

12.6) Have you ever shared information with an uninvolved party out of concern, or warned someone about another person? Was this gossip?

The Appeal of Juicy Morsels of Gossip

The words of a whisperer are like delicious morsels;
they go down into the inner parts of the body. (Proverbs 18:8 and 26:22)

The book of Proverbs talks twice about how appealing whispered words (i.e., gossip) are to those who listen. Gossip sinks into the inner parts of our body. The lure of gossip comes from knowing information that others do not, giving us a sense of importance. It can make us feel better about ourselves to talk about another's problems, but whenever we gossip, we are ingesting poison into the core of our soul.

Questions to Ponder

12.7) How do you relate to these verses from Proverbs?

12.8) Wrong words can backfire and hurt us. Has this ever happened to you? Describe what happened.

What if I Need to Be Advised?

Is it gossip to share with a therapist, pastor, or coach?

There is nothing wrong with seeking advice about a situation in your life that involves other people. The problem comes when you seek advice with an ill motive, or when you seek advice from those who will spread your concern to others. Seek counsel from a trusted friend—one who is fair-minded, understands your strongholds, is not afraid to call out your errors, and will offer you a realistic perspective. You can also ask for advice while keeping the person you're talking about anonymous.

If you solicit the viewpoint of someone you know will always agree with you or popular opinion, you are not requesting advice. Instead, you are venting frustration or seeking to justify yourself, and this is gossip.

Where there is no guidance, a people falls,
but in an abundance of counselors there is safety. (Proverbs 11:14)

Therapists, pastors, sponsors, and coaches should carry no bias toward you or your situation. You should feel safe to share concerns with these people, but no one is perfect. If your most trusted advisors betray your confidence, it is they who are gossiping, not you.

Watch Your Words

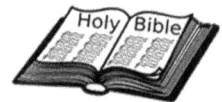

- *"A man who bears false witness against his neighbor is like a war club, or a sword, or a sharp arrow." (Proverbs 25:18)*

- *"A dishonest man spreads strife, and a whisperer separates close friends." (Proverbs 16:28)*

- *"You shall not spread a false report. You shall not join hands with a wicked man to be a malicious witness." (Exodus 23:1)*

- *"You shall not go around as a slanderer among your people, and you shall not stand up against the life of your neighbor: I am the Lord." (Leviticus 19:16)*

- *"Whoever slanders his neighbor secretly I will destroy. Whoever has a haughty look and an arrogant heart I will not endure." (Psalm 101:5)*

Sometimes we do not realize how words we speak come across to others. Pay extra close attention to your words and how people respond to them. Journal what you learn!

Lesson 13 — The Tongue, Part 3

Dealing with People Properly

How do you show love to someone who has hurt or upset you? If possible, you cover over the offense. Go directly to the person in love and help him understand his offense instead of telling others how you were mistreated. Give someone who has offended you the opportunity to make it right.

What if it were you? Would you rather be informed directly if someone has a complaint against you? Would you appreciate it if the person revealed your problem to his friends without ever addressing the issue with you?

People often evade an issue to avoid **conflict**. Avoiding the problem or venting to friends seems easier than coping with the situation. It's easy to believe that once you can "get over it," you can move on, ignoring the problem and never needing to admit your feelings to the one who wronged you. You might avoid conflict, but you do not satisfy your need for justice. As a result, animosity begins to fester.

Whoever covers an offense seeks love, but he who repeats a matter separates close friends. (Proverbs 17:9)

Whoever belittles his neighbor lacks sense, but a man of understanding remains silent. Whoever goes about slandering reveals secrets, but he who is trustworthy in spirit keeps a thing covered. (Proverbs 11:12 – 13)

> ### Question to Ponder
> 13.1) In your experience, what resulted from avoiding conflict?

Conflict

Conflict is beneficial. Without conflict, restoration never happens. Burying a problem creates a larger issue. Over time, pain caused by unresolved offenses turns into anger and resentment.

Conflict resolution is not fighting. People may fear confrontation because they did not learn to engage in effective conflict, modeled in grace and love. Instead, they witnessed disputes handled through argument, belligerence, or brawling. People with shame and insecurity may also avoid conflict, fearing rejection.

> ### Questions to Ponder
> 13.2) Have you ever seen healthy conflict resolution? What did it look like?
> 13.3) How do *you* deal with conflict?

Successful Conflict

It may seem easier to ignore an issue than deal with it, but **a person cannot fix what they do not know is broken.** The easiest and shortest way through an issue is straight ahead. A simple misunderstanding may feel like a major issue until it is addressed. But big problems are quickly solved when those involved can openly and humbly seek resolution. Incorrect handling of a situation (whether that be ignoring it, retaliation, or gossip) compounds the problem.

The Bible teaches us to engage in successful conflict.

1. Search your heart before making a judgment about another person. What angered you? Is a belief or stronghold skewing your perspective of the situation?

   Judge not, that you be not judged. For with the judgment you pronounce you will be judged, and with the measure you use it will be measured to you. (Matthew 7:1 – 2)

2. Talk about your frustration directly with the person involved, not a third party.

   If your brother sins against you, go and tell him his fault, between you and him alone. If he listens to you, you have gained your brother. (Matthew 18:15)

3. Go to the person who has offended you immediately. Don't put it off until later. God wants unresolved conflict handled first, even before giving an offering. Solving problems with others is part of a right relationship with God.

   Be angry and do not sin; do not let the sun go down on your anger, and give no opportunity to the devil. (Ephesians 4:26 – 27)

   So, if you are offering your gift at the altar and there remember that your brother has something against you, leave your gift there before the altar and go. First be reconciled to your brother, and then come and offer your gift. (Matthew 5:23 – 24)

Sowing Discord

You sow discord when, due to your actions or words, a group of people distrust one another, argue, and fight. A person who sows discord plants seeds of discontentment, making others miserable with pessimistic, hateful, or negative attitudes and leading to strife, arguing, and choosing sides.

With perverted heart devises evil, continually sowing discord. (Proverbs 6:14)

> ### Questions to Ponder
> 13.4) Do your pessimistic, negative attitudes prevent you from hearing others or seeking resolution to a problem? In what other ways do you sow discord?
>
> 13.5) In what ways do you strive to make peace?

What If You Cannot Reconcile?

What if someone refuses to hear your grievance or accept your apology? The Scripture says, "As far as it depends on you, live at peace." All you can do is make an honest effort. Do not seek vengeance. God deals with your enemies and can cause your enemies to bless you!

Repay no one evil for evil, but give thought to do what is honorable in the sight of all. If possible, so far as it depends on you, live peaceably with all. Beloved, never avenge yourselves, but leave it to the wrath of God, for it is written, "Vengeance is mine, I will repay, says the Lord."
(Romans 12:17 – 19)

When a man's ways please the Lord, he makes even his enemies to be at peace with him.
(Proverbs 16:7)

Questions to Ponder

13.6) According to the Bible, how should you handle disputes? Will it be easier this way? Why or why not?

13.7) Have you ever solved conflict using these biblical steps? What was the result?

13.8) Has anyone attempted to resolve an issue with you as described in Scripture? How did you respond? Was the situation resolved?

13.9) Are you currently holding anything against someone that needs to be addressed?

13.10) Has anyone ever rejected your efforts to resolve conflict? What was the result?

13.11) What do you consider the most challenging part of handling conflict biblically?

Lesson 14 — The Tongue, Part 4

Inappropriate and Appropriate Talk

Scripture mentions several inappropriate ways in which we use our mouths. One is dirty humor and crude comments. When we are flowing from God's Spirit, we speak what is right. When living out of our flesh, however, we speak harsh words, swear, argue, quarrel, gossip, lie, and so on. Guard your tongue! **Defer your thoughts** to the Lord before speaking. Let His Spirit show you **when to speak** and **when to be silent**.

> *Let there be no filthiness nor foolish talk nor crude joking, which are out of place, but instead let there be thanksgiving.* (Ephesians 5:4)

> *But now you must put them all away: anger, wrath, malice, slander, and obscene talk from your mouth.* (Colossians 3:8)

> *The lips of the righteous know what is acceptable, but the mouth of the wicked, what is perverse.* (Proverbs 10:32)

What Should You Say?

- Use words that are appropriate and full of grace.
  "Let no corrupting talk come out of your mouths, but only such as is good for building up, as fits the occasion, that it may give grace to those who hear." (Ephesians 4:29)

- Your speech should preserve what is good and right, like salt preserves meat. You should give answers full of grace and love, not wrath.
  "Let your speech always be gracious, seasoned with salt, so that you may know how you ought to answer each person." (Colossians 4:6)

- Discuss what is fitting to encourage and help others.
  "A word fitly spoken is like apples of gold in a setting of silver." (Proverbs 25:11)

- Encourage and build up others with your words.
  "Therefore encourage one another and build one another up, just as you are doing." (1 Thessalonians 5:11)

- Give straightforward, honest, yes or no answers.
  "But above all, my brothers, do not swear, either by heaven or by earth or by any other oath, but let your "yes" be yes and your "no" be no, so that you may not fall under condemnation." (James 5:12)

- Pray with gratitude and thanksgiving. Make intercessions for others to lead godly lives.
  "First of all, then, I urge that supplications, prayers, intercessions, and thanksgivings be made for all people, for kings and all who are in high positions, that we may lead a peaceful and quiet life, godly and dignified in every way." (1 Timothy 2:1 – 15)

- Speak truth. *"Therefore, having put away falsehood, let each one of you speak the truth with his neighbor, for we are members one of another."* (Ephesians 4:25)

- Praise others, not yourself. *"Let another praise you, and not your own mouth; a stranger, and not your own lips."* (Proverbs 27:2)

Questions to Ponder

14.1) What circumstances cause you to struggle with inappropriate words?

14.2) How well do you use life-giving words? Can you improve?

Consequences of the Tongue

- *"You shall not take the name of the Lord your God in vain, for the Lord will not hold him guiltless who takes his name in vain. (Exodus 20:7)*

- *"Remind them of these things and charge them before God not to quarrel about words, which does no good, but only ruins the hearers." (2 Timothy 2:14)*

- *"There is one whose rash words are like sword thrusts, but the tongue of the wise brings healing." (Proverbs 12:18)*

- *"A soft answer turns away wrath, but a harsh word stirs up anger." (Proverbs 15:1)*

- *"A gentle tongue is a tree of life, but perverseness in it breaks the spirit." (Proverbs 15:4)*

- *"The words of a wise man's mouth win him favor, but the lips of a fool consume him. The beginning of the words of his mouth is foolishness, and the end of his talk is evil madness." (Ecclesiastes 10:12-13)*

- *"The lips of the righteous feed many, but fools die for lack of sense." (Proverbs 10:21)*

- *"If anyone thinks he is religious and does not bridle his tongue but deceives his heart, this person's religion is worthless." (James 1:26)*

Congratulations!
You have completed the heart check on the tongue!

Questions to Ponder

14.3) Review your answers from all the lessons on the tongue and write down anything you do well.

14.4) Write about any areas discussed in the lessons on the tongue where you need to improve.

14.5) How do you feel about this heart check?

Lesson 15 — Your Thoughts, Part 1

Test Your Heart by Knowing Your Thoughts

You can test your heart by examining the secret thoughts you never reveal to anyone or even those thoughts you refuse to acknowledge. Thoughts invoke feelings and desires. Therefore, what we feel, think, and desire (our "will") displays the core condition of our heart.

Search me, O God, and know my heart! Try me and know my thoughts! (Psalm 139:23)

Questions to Ponder

15.1) **What thoughts have you kept secret? Seek the Lord and ask Him to reveal thoughts you struggle to acknowledge or refuse to admit, even to yourself. List them to bring them into the light.**

15.2) **How do your secret thoughts affect your life? (Consider your emotions, actions, etc.)**

Renew Your Mind

Feelings often direct our conscious thoughts. Changing our thoughts can alter the way we feel and what we desire. Different thinking can override negative emotions. Science has shown that, as our thinking changes, the make-up of our brain changes. The renewal of the mind spoken of in Scripture is the process of replacing poisonous patterns of thinking.

Do not be conformed to this world, <u>but be transformed by the renewal of your mind</u>, that by testing you may discern what is the will of God, what is good and acceptable and perfect. (Romans 12:2)

God's transformation changes how we think. We hear two conflicting reports throughout our lives: lies of the enemy leading to death, or to the true report of the Lord, which leads to life. We choose which one we listen to. Believe the report of the Lord. Choose life and live!

I call heaven and earth to witness against you today, that I have set before you life and death, blessing and curse. Therefore choose life, that you and your offspring may live. (Deuteronomy 30:19)

Our minds require renewal. Without the Lord, our thoughts turn to evil and become enslaved to our flesh.

The LORD saw that the wickedness of man was great in the earth, and that <u>every intention</u> of the <u>thoughts of his heart</u> was only evil continually. (Genesis 6:5)

Therefore, we must guard our minds from the enemy's lies and wrong thinking by keeping our mind focused on the Lord. We must take our thoughts captive, controlling what we allow our mind to absorb.

Set your minds on things that are above, not on things that are on earth. (Colossians 3:2)

You keep him in perfect peace whose mind is stayed on you, because he trusts in you. (Isaiah 26:3)

We destroy speculations and every lofty thing raised up against the knowledge of God, and we take every thought captive to the obedience of Christ. (2 Corinthians 10:5)

How do you take your thoughts captive?

➤ Keep your mind focused on what is good and worthy of praise.

"Finally, brothers, whatever is true, whatever is honorable, whatever is just, whatever is pure, whatever is lovely, whatever is commendable, if there is any excellence, if there is anything worthy of praise, think about these things." (Philippians 4:8)

➤ Guard what goes into your mind. This may include videos, books, or music. Keep your eyes from wicked things that may "cling to you" or have a lasting impact.

"I will not set before my eyes anything that is worthless. I hate the work of those who fall away; it shall not cling to me. (Psalm 101:3)

➤ Set your mind on furthering God's Kingdom and seeking the will of God. Do not become preoccupied by worldly things. The priorities and motivations of this world are not the same priorities and motivations that move a person seeking after God's heart.

"But he turned and said to Peter, 'Get behind me, Satan! You are a hindrance to me. For you are not setting your mind on the things of God, but on the things of man.'" (Matthew 16:23)

"As we look not to the things that are seen but to the things that are unseen. For the things that are seen are transient, but the things that are unseen are eternal." (2 Corinthians 4:18)

"For to set the mind on the flesh is death, but to set the mind on the Spirit is life and peace. For the mind that is set on the flesh is hostile to God, for it does not submit to God's law; indeed, it cannot. Those who are in the flesh cannot please God." (Romans 8:6 – 8)

➤ Do not lean on your own understanding. Instead, seek God, and He will keep you on the right path. There is no fear when we trust in the Lord. Our emotions, senses, and experiences blind us to truth when filtered through our strongholds—the protection responses created by our life experiences. We know truth by God's wise counsel.

"Trust in the Lord with all your heart, and do not lean on your own understanding. In all your ways acknowledge Him, and He will make your paths straight. Do not be wise in your own eyes." (Proverbs 3:5 – 7)

"Seek after the Lord always. With my whole heart I seek you; let me not wander from your commandments!" (Psalm 119:10)

"He is not afraid of bad news; his heart is firm, trusting in the Lord." (Psalm 112:7)

Questions to Ponder

15.3) How have you tried to take your thoughts captive in the past?

15.4) Do you base your judgments and choices on what you think happened without knowing all the facts? Give examples.

15.5) Do you tend to focus more on the positive or negative? List the ways your thoughts focus on the negative.

15.6) What impact does your negativity have on you?

15.7) For each negative thought you mentioned, how can you change to more positive thoughts?

15.8) What do you allow to influence your mind? (TV, movies, books, friends, etc.)

15.9) How do things you watch, read, and hear "cling" to you?

15.10) What should you stop watching, reading, and hearing?

Lesson 16 — Your Thoughts, Part 2

Priorities Are Thoughts That Define Our Heart

We invest in our heart's desire, but our treasure is more than monetary. We treasure time, perhaps to a greater extent than we value money. How many times have you paid extra for a timesaving convenience? Money is replaceable, but time spent is lost forever. Time is our greatest treasure.

For where your treasure is, there will your heart be also. (Luke 12:34)

To understand what your heart most values, examine how you spend your time and why. We make many plans for our time, but the Lord directs the steps of a believer. How do you manage your time? Do you stay busy and use time wisely? Is your time spent in a manner pleasing to the Lord?

Look carefully then how you walk, not as unwise. but as wise, making the best use of the time, because the days are evil. Therefore do not be foolish, but understand what the will of the Lord is. (Ephesians 5:15 – 17)

The heart of man plans his way, but the Lord establishes his steps. (Proverbs 16:9)

Questions to Ponder

16.1) **Prioritize the following list according to their importance to you.**
(1 being the most important and 14 being the least important)

___Career/School   ___Video Games

___Family   ___Social Media

___Friends   ___Prayer/Worship (*Relationship w/God*)

___Extended Family   ___Read/Study Bible

___Finances/Planning   ___House Cleaning/Yard Work

___Television/Music/Reading   ___Serving others/Evangelism

___Entertainment/Dining Out   ___Church Services/Functions

16.2) **We often allow unimportant things to take priority in our lives. Examine your priority list. Write the approximate time you spend with each item on the list in a typical week.**

16.3) **Is the time you spend appropriate for the priority you place on it?**

16.4) **How would God prioritize this list?**

16.5) **To which priorities should you give more or less time?**

Priorities According to the Word

God's Word clearly defines what our top priority should be: God comes first. Why is it so difficult for us Christians to give God precedence? We live in a world full of distractions that absorb our time. Our responsibilities and people's expectations constantly demand our attention. In addition, our own desires vie for our time. God does not want us to abandon our hobbies or interests, but He expects to be our first love. Is your relationship with God first on your priority list?

Consider the following scriptures and reexamine your priorities.

> *"And whatever you do, in word or deed, do everything in the name of the Lord Jesus, giving thanks to God the Father through him." (Colossians 3:17)*

> *"But seek first the kingdom of God and his righteousness, and all these things will be added to you." (Matthew 6:33)*

> *"For what does it profit a man to gain the whole world and forfeit his soul? For what can a man give in return for his soul?" (Mark 8:36 – 37)*

> *"So flee youthful passions and pursue righteousness, faith, love, and peace, along with those who call on the Lord from a pure heart." (2 Timothy 2:22)*

> *"For while bodily training is of some value, godliness is of value in every way, as it holds promise for the present life and also for the life to come." (1 Timothy 4:8)*

> *'Whoever loves father or mother more than me is not worthy of me, and whoever loves son or daughter more than me is not worthy of me." (Matthew 10:37)*

Questions to Ponder

16.6) What distractions prevent you from spending time with the Lord?

16.7) Is your focus more on worldly or heavenly things? How so?

16.8) Are you trusting God with your time? Explain.

16.9) Consider changing your priorities. How do you want your priorities to look?

Lesson 17 — Your Thoughts, Part 3

Searching Your Heart by the Word of God: The Bible Is Your Mirror

To take our thoughts captive to the obedience of Christ is to examine them in the light of God's Word. When you read the Bible, it is like looking in a mirror. As you read, Scripture exposes your thoughts and feelings, showing you the truth about yourself. In this way, **Scripture helps you know your heart as God sees it**. However, **if you are not open** to accepting the truth you find, **God's truth cannot change your life**.

For the word of God is living and active, sharper than any two-edged sword, piercing to the division of soul and of spirit, of joints and of marrow, and discerning the thoughts and intentions of the heart. (Hebrews 4:12)

Our thoughts, feelings, and actions work together to display our heart's condition. We filter messages from people, media, the internet, or other sources through our worldview.

Your **worldview** comprises your preconceived ideas about **how the world is**. Your **philosophy** is your belief about **what life should be** based on past teachings, experiences, fears, and strongholds. As if seeing the world through tinted glasses, we view new information from the perspective created by our philosophy and worldview.

Like anything else, we can filter Scripture through past teaching, our worldview, fears, and strongholds. Therefore, it is important to **ask the Lord for understanding** every time we read His Word, and to **keep an open mind to anything God wants to say**. He will show us truth, but we will derive no good from it if we refuse to listen.

Pray that God will show you the condition of your heart as you read the following passages of Scripture and consider what this means for you.

Everyone who hates his brother is a murderer, and you know that no murderer has eternal life abiding in him. (1 John 3:15)

If anyone says, "I love God," and hates his brother, he is a liar; for he who does not love his brother whom he has seen cannot love God whom he has not seen. (1 John 4:20)

Whoever says he is in the light and hates his brother is still in darkness. (1 John 2:9)

Question to Ponder

17.1) Do you hold hatred in your heart toward another? (These passages are referring not only to a biological brother, but to another in Christ.)

Doing wrong is like a joke to a fool, but wisdom is pleasure to a man of understanding.
(Proverbs 10:23)

Question to Ponder

17.2) Do you ever perceive something wrong as being funny? (Include things from TV, the Internet, movies, social media, and other entertainment sources.)

Love is patient and kind; love does not envy or boast; it is not arrogant or rude. It does not insist on its own way; it is not irritable or resentful. (1 Corinthians 13:4 – 5)

Questions to Ponder

17.3) When do you struggle with patience and kindness?

17.4) Do you envy anyone (desiring what they have)?

17.5) Do you boast about your possessions, your experiences, or your successes? Do you make sure other people can see your possessions or successes (boasting without words)? Explain.

17.6) Do you need to be in control or insist on getting your way? How do you do this?

17.7) What ways do you assume you know better than others?

17.8) List the causes of your irritability or resentments.

For although they knew God, they did not honor him as God or give thanks to him, but they became futile in their thinking, and their foolish hearts were darkened. (Romans 1:21)

Questions to Ponder

17.9) Consider what you grumbled or complained about today, or this week. What complaints are expressed in your words or hidden in your heart?

17.10) List everything for which you can thank God. Take a minute to tell God how thankful you are!

Complaining is a selfish behavior, focusing on a desired outcome and disregarding the reality of a situation. It is a mindset blinded to alternative possibilities. It discounts the desires or needs of others and ignores the blessings God gives in the wake of hard trials. People with a mentality bent on grumbling pay little attention to the good surrounding them. They focus on everything that is not "right" or "fair" in the world, and they discount people's good qualities, instead fixating on their flaws.

Questions to Ponder

17.11) How do you fail to notice positive things and dwell on the negative?

17.12) Consider the situations you grumble about. How are your complaints discounting God's work or nature?

And he said to him, "You shall love the Lord your God with all your heart and with all your soul and with all your mind." (Matthew 22:37)

Questions to Ponder

17.13) Do you apply the command to "love God with all your heart, mind, and soul" in your life? How would you like to do so?

Lesson 18 — Your Thoughts, Part 4

Motives

Motives are the intentions or reasons behind our choices. Sometimes we do the right thing with ill motives. Perhaps our motives are honorable, but our actions result in an unintended outcome. Many times we are unaware, or refuse to consider, the motives that dwell in our subconscious thoughts. We need to examine the motives behind our thoughts, words, actions, and even our prayers.

Thoughts and motives interlink. Our thoughts influence our motives, and our motives influence our thoughts, which direct our decisions. Thoughts and ideas filtered through fear, insecurity, selfishness, and our individual versions of right and wrong give birth to wrong, selfish motives. **Regardless of the outcome, it is the heart's intent that matters to God.** Doing good things with wicked intention is sin. And when our heart's motives line up with God's ways, mistakes resulting in a negative outcome are not always sinful. God examines the spirit in which we act. He does **not condemn** us for **honest mistakes** when we strive to be obedient to His Word.

Repent, therefore, of this wickedness of yours, and pray to the Lord that,
if possible, the intent of your heart may be forgiven you. (Acts 8:22)

Questions to Ponder

18.1) Define in your own words which intentions of your heart please the Lord, and which motives He would consider wickedness.

18.2) How do your motives influence your thoughts, ideas, decisions, or actions?

Influence

Be careful with whom you associate. Everything you see and hear influences your thoughts, and the people in your life are your greatest influence. Your spouse and close friendships should have similar values and beliefs to yours. It is difficult, sometimes painful, and often detrimental when your close relationships oppose your faith. Scripture calls this being **unequally yoked**.

If your friends are not of moral character, you will pick up more of their bad habits than they will pick up of your good ones. You may keep your core values, but people do affect how you think. Are you a people pleaser? Your desire for approval affects your motives. Guarding your mind includes guarding which influences you allow in.

Do two walk together, unless they have agreed to meet?
(Amos 3:3)

The fear of man lays a snare, but whoever trusts in the Lord is safe.
(Proverbs 29:25)

18.3) Do you keep company with people of godly character?

18.4) Do you compromise your values or change your behavior when with certain people?

18.5) Do you behave in certain ways to be accepted or to avoid another's judgment?

Emotions

Our emotions often speak louder than our thoughts. Thoughts are the place where our emotions dwell. Emotions develop as our minds interpret situations through our conscious thoughts, memories, and beliefs. This is how our emotions can help us understand our unconscious thoughts. **When you discover the thought behind an emotion, you discover what is in your heart, which helps you understand your expectations and sort through your motives.**

In the **conscious mind,** the part of the mind in which we are currently aware and process our thoughts, it is easy to connect a thought to the emotion it evokes. For example, if someone cuts you off in traffic, you think, "They almost caused a wreck!" and you experience fear. Your fear connects to your realization that you almost wrecked your car.

Have you ever experienced an emotion, like sadness or fear, that seems to have no origin? Thoughts buried in the **unconscious mind** can trigger an emotional response that seems illogical or out of place, like experiencing sudden fear or sadness when you step outside.

Think of your brain as a personal computer. Every thought, emotion, memory, and belief becomes a file stored on the hard drive of your brain. The **conscious mind** is like your open, active files. The **subconscious mind** is like your file storage, which gives you easy access to thoughts, knowledge, and emotions, which your conscious mind may pull up as needed.

Once the conscious mind processes a thought, it files it in a directory called memory in the **unconscious mind.** If the mind believes the thought is accurate knowledge, it stores it as a **belief.** Your brain automatically files every thought, emotion, belief, and memory. While your mind is assimilating current experiences, it is running scans of all your stored files, seeking relevant information.

If an **unconscious process** of your brain triggers an emotional response, your conscious mind will know the emotion, but it may not be aware of the reason for it. This is when **you must step back and learn what your emotions are telling you.**

Toxic Emotions or Toxic Thoughts?

Emotions **can inform you** of your thoughts, but they **should** *never* **guide** your decisions. Even though they generate powerful feelings, **emotions have no ability to decipher between right and wrong.** Emotions are neither good nor bad, but if they develop from strongholds and wrong thinking, they can deceive you or control you.

Not all emotions that feel bad are toxic. Grief feels bad, but the message grief portrays is deep love for another. People only grieve for what they love. **Toxic emotions are emotions that trap you or feed your flesh's sin nature, drawing you away from God or people.** Envy feeds the sin of lust or jealousy can cause dissention. Fear can be a healthy emotion that protects you from danger, or it can become toxic, crippling you from making positive changes in your life.

What determines whether an emotion is healthy or toxic, is the message or thought behind it and your response to it. For example, anger shows a real or perceived injustice; it is neither positive nor negative. However, your response to anger may be considered either good or evil. We can allow anger to fester into hate or use the information it gives us to resolve a conflict and forgive another person.

It is thoughts, not emotions, which are healthy or destructive. Therefore, it is vital to determine the truth about your thoughts. This keeps your heart in right standing with the Lord and prevents your flesh from using your emotions to trigger sin.

It may be difficult to identify the thought causing a certain emotion. Think about **what happened before you felt it. Are you feeling another emotion as well? What are you thinking now? Does this emotion feel like something you have experienced in the past?** Answering these questions can help you discover whether the feeling is rational or based on a lie.

Do not confuse thoughts with feelings. We can express feelings in one or two words, but if you need a sentence to express a feeling, you are likely sharing a thought. "I feel like I don't deserve love" is a thought, not an emotion. "I feel shame," on the other hand, expresses an emotion.

Questions to Ponder

18.6) How well do you handle your emotions? Explain.

18.7) Do you feel emotions which seem to have no cause? Explain.

18.8) Pay attention to your emotions this week. Using the questions in bold above, examine the thoughts behind each emotion. Are these toxic or healthy thoughts?

18.9) Were you unable to identify the underlying thought of an emotion? Describe the emotion and the circumstances surrounding it.

Congratulations!
You have completed the heart check on your thoughts!

Questions to Ponder

18.10) Review all your answers from the lessons on thoughts and write down any ways in which you do well.

18.11) Write about any areas discussed in the lessons on thoughts where you need to improve.

18.12) How do you feel about this heart check?

Lesson 19 — Your Actions, Part 1

Actions

Your actions show the condition of your heart. Situations lead to thoughts, which result in actions. Examine your actions to discover the feelings and thoughts that triggered the action. We must know why we behave as we do to understand and guard our hearts.

Above all else, guard your heart, for everything you do flows from it. (Proverbs 4:23)

We invest our time, money, and attention in what we treasure.

Integrity

If your words say one thing but your actions say another, you are disingenuous. Scripture says to let your words be simply "yes" or "no" (see Matthew 5:37), referring to your integrity. Your word alone should be as dependable as a vow. Consider this parable:

"But what do you think? A man had two sons. And he went to the first and said, 'Son, go and work in the vineyard today.' And he answered, 'I will not,' but afterward he changed his mind and went. And he went to the other son and said the same. And he answered, 'I go, sir, 'but did not go. Which of the two did the will of his father?" They said, "The first." Jesus said to them, "Truly, I say to you, the tax collectors and the prostitutes go into the kingdom of God before you. For John came to you in the way of righteousness, and you did not believe him, but the tax collectors and the prostitutes believed him. And even when you saw it, you did not afterward change your minds and believe him."
(Matthew 21:28 – 32)

Questions to Ponder

19.1) How do the things you say differ from your genuine feelings and actions?

19.2) Do you ever give into laziness, avoid work, or make excuses?

This parable applies to every life situation. If our words say one thing but our actions say the opposite, we are not trustworthy. We see this lack of integrity in **the masks** we wear for certain people, **lies** we tell to fit in, **excuses** made to avoid work, and **claiming to** believe or like something to gain approval. In every case, our actions do not match our words or what is really in our heart. When this happens, we are not being honest.

Who is wise and understanding among you? By his good conduct let him show his works in the meekness of wisdom. But if you have bitter jealousy and selfish ambition in your hearts, do not boast and be false to the truth. This is not the wisdom that comes down from above, but is earthly, unspiritual, demonic. For where jealousy and selfish ambition exist, there will be disorder and every vile practice. But the wisdom from above is first pure, then peaceable, gentle, open to reason, full of mercy and good fruits, impartial and sincere. And a harvest of righteousness is sown in peace by those who make peace. (James 3:13 – 18)

<u>Questions to Ponder</u>

19.3) Jealousy and selfish ambition (seeking to acquire success at the expense of another) produce disorder and vile actions. How have your jealousy or ambition become harmful?

19.4) True wisdom comes from good motives and leads to peace, mercy, reasonableness, and other good actions. Describe the positive result of your good conduct?

So, whether you eat or drink, or whatever you do, do all to the glory of God.
(1 Corinthians 10:31)

<u>Question to Ponder</u>

19.5) We are told to glorify God in everything we do, even the little things! In what ways do your actions glorify God?

Scripture speaks of "numbering our days." This refers to our brief existence on earth compared to eternity. As we consider our limited number of days, we make what we do in those days count, and choose not to waste any time.

Who considers the power of your anger, and your wrath according to the fear of you?
So teach us to number our days that we may get a heart of wisdom. (Psalm 90:11 – 12)

<u>Questions to Ponder</u>

19.6) How much time do you spend on self-gratifying or trivial activities?

19.7) What activities do you consider a waste of time?

19.8) How do you expect the Lord wants you to use your time?

How you invest your money and possessions is a powerful statement to the condition of your heart. It displays either your love for God and people or your level of greed. God wants you to give from the genuine desire of your heart, not just because it is the "right thing to do."

Generosity goes further than giving stuff. Often the most valuable gift we can give to another is our time and our ear. Good listeners support and encourage others. Giving your time is a genuine display of love and kindness to a person and service to the Lord.

Each one must give as he has decided in his heart, not reluctantly or under compulsion,
for God loves a cheerful giver. (2 Corinthians 9:7)

Sell your possessions and give to the needy. Provide yourselves with moneybags that do not grow old, with a treasure in the heavens that does not fail, where no thief approaches and no moth destroys. For where your treasure is, there will your heart be also.
(Luke 12:33 – 34)

No servant can serve two masters, for either he will hate the one and love the other, or he will be devoted to the one and despise the other. You cannot serve God and money. (Luke 16:13)

Questions to Ponder

19.9) In what do you invest a significant amount of money?

19.10) If your spending does not represent your treasure, what changes must you make?

19.11) Do you hold your possessions with a firm grip, or are you open to giving them away if the situation calls for it? What are you unwilling to let go?

19.12) You invest your time and attention in what you treasure. Are you quick to give time to others? Why or why not?

19.13) Are you attentive when listening to others? Do you let other things—the time, your phone, or a squirrel outside—distract you?

Lesson 20 — Your Actions, Part 2

Read the Scriptures and Answer the Questions

Be angry, and do not sin; ponder in your own hearts on your beds, and be silent. (Psalm 4:4)

Questions to Ponder

20.1) List all the ways your anger causes you to sin.

20.2) Do you say words you should not say, or words you regret out of anger?

20.3) How do you control your angry responses?

20.4) What makes you angry? Does your anger come because you were hurt, fearful, or desire something you cannot get? Is your anger because of an injustice?

The wise of heart will receive commandments, but a babbling fool will come to ruin.
(Proverbs 10:8)

Questions to Ponder

20.5) How well do you receive correction? Be honest: Do you place blame on others?

20.6) How do you respond to rules or when confronted?

20.7) Do you listen more than you speak? How well do you hear others?

20.8) Does your opinion matter, and to whom?

20.9) Do you talk over others or talk a lot because you feel people do not hear or value what you say?

The heart is deceitful above all things, and desperately sick; who can understand it?
"I the Lord search the heart and test the mind, to give every man according to his ways, according to the fruit of his deeds." (Jeremiah 17:9 – 10)

Question to Ponder

20.10) Pray and ask the Lord to search your heart and test your mind and actions. What has He revealed to you?

Congratulations!
You have completed the heart check on your actions!

Questions to Ponder

20.11) Review all your answers from the actions lessons and write down any areas you do well.

20.12) Write down all areas from the action lessons where you need improvement.

20.13) How do you feel about this heart check? *(Continue to next page)*

Now What?

For this people's heart has grown dull, and with their ears they can barely hear, and their eyes they have closed; lest they should see with their eyes and hear with their ears and understand with their heart and turn, and I would heal them. (Acts 28:27)

Do not be discouraged by a negative answer in your heart check. Do not worry; this does not mean you are a bad person or beyond hope. Your heart check was never intended to condemn you, but to expose areas of your flesh that hinder you. Do not be disappointed with yourself, thinking, "So much is wrong with me." Everyone has wrong thoughts and desires, and everyone acts on them sometimes. You will soon discover that those things **do not define you**.

The solution is seeking the Lord and repenting when He points out an issue. Refusing to examine or repent from an issue may harden your heart, which creates a dull, cold, miserable person. However, if you bring your flaws into the open, God removes them. Don't expect all your flaws to change at once, either; this will only overwhelm you. Transformation is a lifelong process. Give your sin to God and let Him make you into His image!

Repentance

What does it mean to repent? Repentance is not just saying you are sorry. Many people believe that if you say you are sorry and really mean it, then all is forgiven, and you can move forward. It is true, you must sincerely apologize, but repentance is not moving forward. It is turning around. It is turning from your sin to head in the opposite direction, back to God.

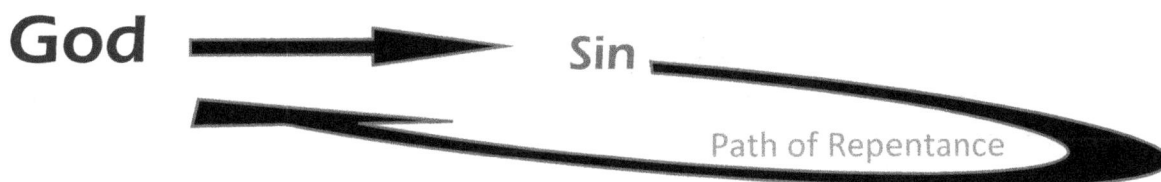

God → Sin — Path of Repentance

Questions to Ponder

20.14) Go back through your answers at the end of each heart check section. Write down the areas for improvement that you mentioned in each one.

20.15) Change is a process that takes time. To start that process, repent.

- Make a conscious decision to change each one of these things and ask for the Lord's forgiveness where needed.
- Pray. Tell God your desire to repent and ask Him to change your heart!
- Write what you think about your choice. Do you believe that God will change your heart as you desire?

20.16) Use the worksheet on the next page to create some goals you wish to work toward with the Lord.

Making a "Heart Check Plan"

Putting the Pieces Together

You have come a long way by recognizing the condition of your heart. Here is the good news: The areas that need improving do not define who you are! Every person has some things in their heart that need to be changed or that they wish were different. You have likely discovered some of these things in yourself. You have also seen the good in your heart, such as times you have shown compassion, used words to encourage, and so on.

What do you do with this information? The first step is to understand exactly what needs to be corrected and the person you desire to become. As your journey continues, you will discover the root of your heart issues. You will see how it is possible for the Lord to transform you into the person He created you to be, and you will learn to keep your heart in check to prevent falling back into old ways.

Directions:

List the things you wish to change, and the result you wish to see.
You may copy this page or write the lists in your journal.

List the areas you wish to change.

_____
_____
_____
_____
_____
_____
_____
_____
_____
_____
_____
_____
_____
_____
_____
_____
_____
_____
_____
_____

For each change, write the desired result.

_____
_____
_____
_____
_____
_____
_____
_____
_____
_____
_____
_____
_____
_____
_____
_____
_____
_____
_____
_____

What do you feel is (are) your most damaging issue(s)?

_____
_____
_____
_____

Questions to Ponder

20.17) Reference the "Making a Heart Check Plan" worksheet.
For each change you want to see, write a scripture that encourages you towards making that change.

* Start by focusing on your most damaging issue.

* Memorize the verse for the issue you are addressing.

* When you struggle with the issue, consider the verse and journal.

* Do not attempt to solve every issue at once. Allow the Lord to guide you.

Lesson 21 — Take Inventory of Your Life

Now that you know what is in your heart, it is time to investigate where it originated. We start life with a sin nature; that means we have a tendency toward sin. However, it is our experiences that bring about fear, anger, depression, loneliness, insecurity, shame, and so on. These are the root causes of most addictions, codependency, and destructive behaviors.

The First Step

The first step of your inventory prepares your mind to examine past hurts. For some people, the pain of their past causes blocked or denied emotions. This makes it difficult to be honest about the experiences associated with that pain. Your heart check was a good starting point. Examine your answers and find clues that show your feelings.

Invest yourself in the following questions. **Take your time and give thorough answers.** When you feel as if you have found every answer, ask yourself, "What else?" Continue to seek what else you can add until you have completely exhausted all possibilities.

> ### First Step Questions
>
> 21.1) What things anger you? (Past experiences, loss, missed opportunities, abuse, etc.)
>
> 21.2) What are your fears? (People, Illness, rejection, loss, failure, abandonment, opinions, the future, etc.)
>
> 21.3) What do you feel guilty about? Why do you feel shame?
>
> 21.4) Are you honest? Do you make excuses and feel like a victim (self-pity), or blame others for your faults?

The Second Step

Everything so far has prepared you for your inventory. This is a tremendous step toward changing the bad thinking behind the destructive behaviors and addictions that rule your life, but it can be a difficult process. Completing your inventory will help you identify the negative messages that shaped your self-image and behaviors, and teach you beneficial ways to think about your life. Thinking differently can change the impact of painful life events.

In Step Two, you will list significant events in your life. If you avoid thinking about certain times in life or have difficulty acknowledging painful words and circumstances, this step may seem overwhelming or frightening. Admitting your poor choices and the pain others have caused you can be painful and embarrassing. Do not get stuck in these feelings. Trust God and your coach to get you through.

➤ Realize you are safe. Your coach experienced his own situations that left similar scars on his heart. His experience may not be the same, but he understands pain and shame. Your coach will not judge or condemn you.

➤ Remember gratitude. Think how far you have already come. Remember all the Lord has done and trust He will never leave you. Remember that praise is the key that unlocks your freedom.

Instructions for the Step Two Worksheet

Carefully read the following instructions before beginning.

The Step Two Worksheet will guide you through your life inventory. *Remembering back as far as possible, list every **significant** event in your life. Be as honest and thorough as possible. **Trying to remember what happened in your life can be difficult.** It helps to consider your life in seasons and groups (i.e., family, school, college, marriage, significant friendships, work relationships, and so on).*

- Start by listing just the events leaving out details, messages, or emotions related to the situation.
- After completing every list on the worksheet, write causes for each item on each list.
- Then go back through your lists again and write the messages for each item on each list.

What are messages?

After writing each list (and causes), you will write the messages received from the situation you listed. A "message" is the impression left on your heart from others' words or actions (whether or not the person intended to imply the message by their words or actions). How did the situation speak into your life or about your character and worth? Hidden messages significantly influence how you view yourself.

For example: Your aunt tells you, "You are just like your father." If your father is a brilliant, moral, successful man, the message you receive would be affirming. However, if your father was a drunk and absent from your life, the unspoken message you hear might be, "I will never amount to anything" or "I am rejected, worthless." In this case, the root of the message is your opinion of your father. Your aunt may have noticed something that resembled a positive trait or talent your father has, but you hear her words filtered through your own pre-conceived ideas about him.

How to identify significant events

List people and/or situations that occurred during major life events, trials, or addiction. Include any event related to an issue you recognize. Think about the answers you wrote to the questions in Step One. What life situations are related to or impacted by those feelings? (For example, if you have an intense fear of rejection, include situations in which you felt left out or ridiculed.)

List any situation or comment that reinforced a destructive message. (For instance, someone saying you are an unwanted child seems insignificant but reinforces the message that you are not loveable.) Any comment that still sticks out in your mind is significant. You may add to your lists anytime during this step as you remember relative situations.

Step Two Tips

➤ The inventory is the most intensive part of this journey. Clear your schedule of unimportant or distracting things during this time. Allow life to slow down for a few weeks.

➤ **Do not begin your inventory during a major life event. This is not a good time to grow a family, get married, get a new job, go on a family vacation, or plan a move.**

➤ Set aside time each day to work until your inventory is complete.

➤ When making your lists, skip a line between each situation or person so you can add more information later.

➤ Be honest. Do not leave out an event, person, or situation because it is difficult. You are safe to express these things

➤ Give only enough information to trigger your recollection of the event, people, etc.

➤ It is okay to mention the same person on multiple lists or in several events.

Step Two Worksheet

Use the guide below to list the significant circumstances in your life. Bring any questions to your coach. Keep the descriptions of the events mentioned brief.

Inventory Lists: **From your youngest memory to the present day**

Part 1 – Create Six Lists
(You will reference these lists in parts 2 and 3 of this worksheet and in Step Three.)

1) List significant people, events, places, or ideas that had a positive impact in your life.

2) List people, situations, or ideas that you resent. (Resentment is unresolved fear or anger.)

3) List people, situations, or ideas that hurt you.

4) List situations, people, events, places, or ideas that caused you to fear.

5) List people in which sexual conduct has caused harm to yourself or others.

6) List people *you* have harmed. (Do not include the sexual harms mentioned above.)

Part 2 – Causes and Effects

- Return to List One. Describe the circumstances around the items listed and explain how they affected you positively.

- Return to List Two. Describe the circumstances around the items listed and why they angered you.

- Return to List Three. For each item listed, describe the type of harm you experienced and the cause of your hurt.

- Return to List Four. Describe the circumstances around the items listed and how they caused fear.

- Return to List Five. For each item listed, explain the nature of the sexual conduct and how it caused harm. Note: If you are the victim of rape or abuse, you are not at fault. Write about the harm caused *to* you.

- Return to List Six. Describe the circumstances around the items listed. In what way(s) were you responsible for causing the harm?

Part 3 – Messages

- Go back through *each list*. For each item describe the messages you received from the situation. How did this circumstance affect how you perceive your value and identity? How did it affect your character? How did the situation change your view of another person?

> ➢ KEEP THESE LISTS! You will use them throughout this book!

If you are confused by this step, ask your coach for a sample worksheet.

Lesson 22 — The Third Inventory Step

The Third Step

Completing this step of your inventory will be the most freeing thing you ever do. You will bring the darkness in your life into the light, discover the buried truth behind each secret, confess it all to someone you trust, and release it all to the Lord, removing its power. Light changes our perspective, allowing us to see our life through new eyes.

And I will lead the blind in a way that they do not know, in paths that they have not known I will guide them. I will turn the darkness before them into light, the rough places into level ground. These are the things I do, and I do not forsake them. (Isaiah 42:16)

Instructions for the *Step Three* Rebuilt *Inventory Worksheet*
(You will need your lists from Step Two to complete this step.)

➤ Complete an inventory worksheet for each item in List 2 (resentments) and discuss them with your coach. (Your coach has a resentment activity.)

➤ Complete an inventory worksheet **for each item in Lists 3, 4, and 5** and discuss them with your coach.

➤ After completing every worksheet, your coach will work with you to compare the messages received from all your negative situations with the positive impacts in List 1. You will look for messages with the greatest influence in your life. Which messages speak the loudest in your mind? Which speak truth? Is the truth louder than the lies you believe?

➤ Examine the harms you caused in List 6. Work with your coach to see how strongholds from past experiences and beliefs influenced your actions.

➤ Next, your coach will lead you in an activity to release your past to the Lord, empowering you to move forward. (Keep your lists for additional activities.)

➤ After confessing your lists to the Lord, **let them go! Do not take them back!** A balloon cannot fly away if you hold on to the string!

Step Three Tips

➤ Record your thoughts and feelings before, during, and after the event occurred. Search for triggers and patterns in your thoughts, feelings, or situations

➤ Write your answers to the questions on the second page of the Step Three worksheet in your journal, adding thorough details.

➤ Set aside time daily to work on your inventory. It is the most important part of your journey, so devote your time and effort to it.

➤ **You may** continue **to move forward in this book while working on this step.** The remaining lessons in this book can help you navigate difficult emotions and overcome stuck points.

➤ **Do not worry about how long the inventory takes.** This is **your** journey; it moves at your pace.

➤ Do not move on to the next book until your inventory is completed.

➤ **Keep all your lists!** They will be used for additional activities.

THIS WAY → Your coach has a vital role in this step. He or she will guide you through two life-changing activities. Prepare a full day for each activity.

Step Three — *Rebuilt* Inventory Worksheet

You may make copies of the worksheet or use it as a guide for writing in your journal.

What happened? Describe the circumstance/situation.

_____

_____

Was there an offense? (Did someone wrong me or offend me? Did I wrong or offend someone else?) What was the exact nature of the wrong?

_____

_____

Is the offense real or perceived? What was my part or responsibility in this situation?

_____

_____

Select what triggered your response to the situation. Do/Did you feel:

- ☐ Fearful/Anxious
- ☐ Like a failure
- ☐ Not good enough
- ☐ Unliked/Unloved
- ☐ Rejected or Insecure
- ☐ Vulnerable

- ☐ Angry
- ☐ Defiant/Controlling/Prideful
- ☐ Suspicious
- ☐ Jealous/Envious
- ☐ Bitter/Resentful
- ☐ Threatened (financially, physically, emotionally, etc.)

- ☐ Lonely/Neglected
- ☐ Guilty/Shameful
- ☐ Loss
- ☐ Self-pity (feeling sorry for yourself)

How did I respond to this situation?

_____

_____

_____

Were You:
- ☐ Tired/Exhausted
- ☐ Hungry
- ☐ Hurt emotionally
- ☐ Hurt physically

What harm came from (or could come from) my response to the situation?

_____

_____

_____

_____

Were Your Responses:
- ☐ Selfish/Self-seeking
- ☐ Dishonest
- ☐ Inconsiderate/Lacking Compassion
- ☐ Lacking Self-control/Self-discipline
- ☐ Controlling or Manipulating Others
- ☐ Prideful (Rejecting counsel/ prideful self-reliance)
- ☐ Ambitious for social/relational gain
- ☐ Ambitious for financial gain

How could I have responded differently?

_____

_____

_____

Can I correct the damage caused by my response? *If so, how?*

_____

_____

Answer the questions that correspond with the "Do you feel" boxes you checked.

(For example, if you checked the boxes for anger and insecurity, you would answer the questions under number 1 and number 2 below.)

1. **Angry, bitter, or resentful**
   a) What is the emotion behind the anger?
   b) What are you resentful or bitter about?
   c) What past circumstances have fed into this resentment?

2. **Fearful anxious, insecure, rejected, vulnerable, threatened, suspicious, jealous, envious**
   a) What are you afraid will happen?
   b) What situations in the past have taught you to fear this result?

3. **Self-pity, shameful, guilty, not enough, a failure, unliked, or unloved**
   a) What past experiences are making you feel this way?
   b) Are you being fair to yourself? Is this feeling reasonable or is it self-pity?

4. **Defiance, controlling, prideful**
   a) What were/are you trying to control?
   b) What happened in the past that made you feel a need to control in this circumstance?

5. **Lonely, loss, neglected**
   a) What is missing that causes you to feel this way?
   b) What losses in your past may have fed into this feeling?

_____

_____

_____

_____

_____

_____

To change our behaviors, we must change the way we think about things. When we identify where our patterns of emotion and behavior come from, we can separate the truth from the lies. In the future when we find ourselves in a similar situation, we can think about the truth we have learned and reject the thoughts and feelings that have held us captive.

What are the wrong messages—lies—you are believing in this circumstance?

_____

_____

What truth should you believe?

_____

_____

Chapter Six

Problematic Thinking
& Stuck Points

FRUSTRATION IS A LOCK

PATIENCE IS THE KEY

Not only that, but we rejoice in our sufferings, knowing that suffering produces endurance, and endurance produces character, and character produces hope, and hope does not put us to shame, because God's love has been poured into our hearts through the Holy Spirit who has been given to us. (Romans 5:3-5)

THE LORD IS THE LOCKSMITH, THE MAKER OF EVERY KEY

I am the vine; you are the branches. Whoever abides in me and I in him, he it is that bears much fruit, for apart from me you can do nothing. (John 15:5)

WHAT IS THIS FRUIT?

But the fruit of the Spirit is love, joy, peace, patience, kindness, goodness, faithfulness, gentleness, self-control; against such things there is no law. (Galatians 5:22-23)

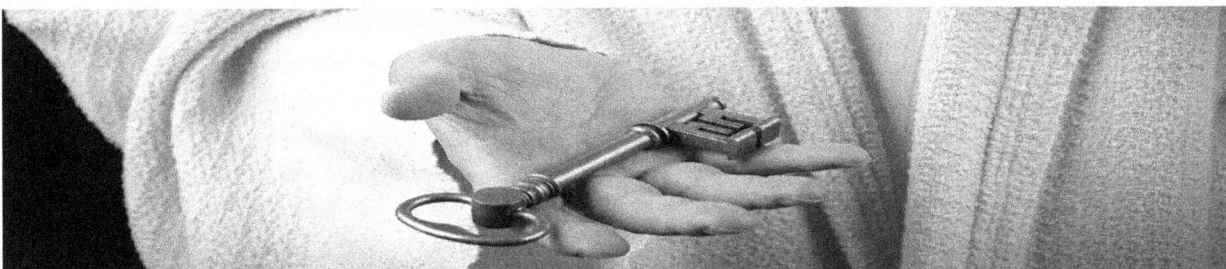

Lesson 23 — Problematic Thinking

Cognitive distortions are irrational, exaggerated patterns of thought that convince our mind to believe something untrue. These thought distortions go beyond simple negativity; **they may solidify a negative thought into a belief.**

There are many ways your thinking can distort your view of yourself, other people, and the world around you. Your ideas may have come from how you learned to relate in childhood, your life experiences, or when your belief system conflicts with the reality you experience. This is natural: Our mind attempts to make sense of what we do not understand and protect us from being hurt.

Some thoughts are automatic responses to an experience. These thoughts often line up with core beliefs about yourself, others, and the world. **Automatic thoughts are like a thinking habit.** You think without knowing you are thinking, and when these thoughts are negative, you may see even a positive event in a negative light. Thoughts that cause shame, bitterness, anger, fear, or insecurity may even lead to symptoms of depression or anxiety.

Check Your Thinking

➢ Read the "Problematic Thinking Patterns" worksheet.

➢ Check your inventory worksheets for thought patterns that may have caused misunderstandings or led to a toxic situation.

➢ This worksheet is not an exhaustive list but provides a good starting point to show the adverse effects that can result from your thinking.

Use the "Problematic Thinking Worksheet" to examine ways you are thinking about your experiences this week.

1. **Watch for yourself or someone else to use one of these thinking patterns and write about it in your journal.**

2. **Look for an example of each type of distorted thinking.**

3. **On the worksheet, check the box next to the thought distortions you notice in yourself.**

Patterns of Problematic Thinking Worksheet

> **What thoughts are keeping you from a full recovery? These are your stuck points thoughts that keep you from forgiving another, or that keep you angry or insecure. Often, these thoughts originate from problematic thinking patterns.**

Directions:

Check the boxes next to a pattern you recognize in yourself and write an example for each checked pattern of how you have seen this pattern in your thinking.

☐ **Fortune-telling** – Jumping to conclusions, predicting or assuming a future outcome, or expecting the worst possible outcome to happen.
Clue words: "What if …" statements.

☐ **Magnifying or Minimizing** – Magnifying is exaggerating a situation or blowing it out of proportion (i.e., making a mountain out of a molehill). Minimizing discounts the importance of something relevant. Often, they work together.
Example: Your team wins a game, but you minimize the win because you missed a goal, and you magnify your failure to get the goal.

☐ **Filtering** – Filtering out either positive or negative information about a situation.
Examples: The attitude that "having integrity won't pay my bills," or ignoring disciplinary action from a boss and only focusing on praise from a coworker (or vice-versa).

☐ **Polarized Thinking** – Oversimplifying things as good/bad, right/wrong. This is also referred to as "black and white" or "all or nothing" thinking. This way of thinking does not acknowledge gray areas or contributing circumstances.
Example: You accuse your spouse of failing to contribute to the family because they did not clean the house—ignoring the fact that your spouse was sick in bed most of the week.

☐ **Overgeneralization** – Drawing a conclusion based on one or two incidents. You perceive an incident as an event that will happen again and again, or as a pattern that will continue forever.
Clue words: "All," "None," "Always," "Never," "Every," "Constantly," "Can't," "Won't."
*Examples: "I **can't** get my bills right, **every** month I am late on something." Or someone cancels plans with you, and now you do not believe you can count on them.*

☐ **Personalization** – Taking what others do personally or comparing yourself with others. This thinking causes you to assume another's actions are a response to you or your behaviors. It may also be taking the blame for things outside of your responsibility or control.
Example: "She did not say anything at the meeting; I must have made her angry." "I should have been able to stop the accident."

- **Labeling** – When a person makes a mistake or something happens you dislike, you label the person, object, or situation based on that experience.
  Examples: "The homework assignment is stupid." "She is so lazy." "I am a failure."

- **Mind-reading** – Assuming the thoughts of others with no evidence of their opinions. This could be an assumption that a person has negative thoughts toward you, or assuming you know why a person acts a certain way.
  Examples: "They will think I am worthless." "He must think I am stupid." "She has no good reason for staying home; she must be hiding something."

- **Emotional Reasoning** – Considering your emotions as proof of the reality of a situation.
  Examples: "I feel fear, so there is danger." "I feel stupid, so I am stupid."

- ***Should* Statements** – Believing if you or someone else did something different, a situation would have had a better outcome. This thinking often places unrealistic expectations on yourself or others and may lead to shame, anger, or bitterness.
  Clue words: "Should," "must," "ought."
  Examples: "I should have known that car was coming." "I should have known I couldn't trust him." "He ought to have more gratitude for everything I did for him."

- **Blaming** – Holding other people responsible for your pain or seeing everything bad as someone else's fault entirely.
  Example: "I tripped because you got in my way."

- **Self-serving Bias** –Believing everything good that happens around you points to your excellent character, but negative events are out of your control.
- *Example: People with this thinking may refuse to admit their flaws and go to great lengths to prove they are not wrong. They may see themselves as always being right, believe their opinions are facts, or fail to consider the opinions or feelings of others*

- **Fallacy of Change** – The expectation that other people will change what they think or do to make you happy. This thinking insists on having its own way and may pressure or manipulate people to enforce it. Your happiness requires that another person change.
  Example: Refusing to eat a meal with the family because you dislike the prepared food.

- **Just World Fallacy** – The assumption that you get what you deserve in life, or that everything must be fair and equal. It is the belief that good things happen to good people, and bad things happen to bad people.
  Examples: "They deserve to live in poverty because they do not work hard enough." "I went out on a date with my coworker because my husband cheated. It's only fair."

Lesson 24 — Stuck Points

I Am Stuck and Cannot Get Past This! What Do I Do?

Why do we get stuck in unpleasant emotions and unhealthy behaviors? We become stuck because of the way we think. Our life experiences form our belief system. We filter everything that happens through that belief system. **Sometimes this filter makes it hard to see the truth.**

Most people have sought the approval of others to validate what they believe. We have a spiritual enemy who lies to us. We leave a door open to receive his lies when the opinions of a parent, spouse, friend, church leader, or anyone other than God shape our identity and worldviews. A person's opinion may seem right, but that does not mean it is truth.

> *There is a way that seems right to a man, but its end is the way to death.*
> *(Proverbs 14:12)*

Let us say, for example, that you have a natural talent and calling in a field. You apply for a job in that field and show proficient understanding of the job. The interviewer calls you back. You did not get the job, because you do not meet their experience requirements. Your mind forms a belief that you are unqualified for this career, and thus you give up seeking that kind of work.

In this situation, the enemy tells you the lie that you are unable—unqualified for this work. You hear the thought as your own and internalize it as a belief. The truth is that God gifted you for that career, and there are other jobs in the field for which you may qualify. However, the doubt and insecurity placed in your heart destroys your confidence. You no longer pursue what God created you to do. In this scenario, man's rejection opened a door for the enemy to frame your thinking in a detrimental way. Your belief that you are not good enough causes you to abandon your calling.

> *For am I now seeking the approval of man, or of God? Or am I trying to please*
> *man? If I were still trying to please man, I would not be a servant of Christ.*
> *(Galatians 1:10)*

> *Because there is no truth in him [the devil]. When he lies, he speaks out of his own*
> *character, for he is a liar and the father of lies.*
> *(John 8:44)*

> *And no wonder, for even Satan disguises himself as an angel of light.*
> *(2 Corinthians 11:14)*

> *But I am afraid that as the serpent deceived Eve by his cunning, your thoughts will*
> *be led astray from a sincere and pure devotion to Christ.*
> *(2 Corinthians 11:3)*

To get unstuck, you must:

> ➤ Recognize what you are thinking and believing
>
> ➤ See how those beliefs affect your emotional state and your actions
>
> ➤ Challenge those thoughts to recognize any lies you believe
>
> ➤ Submit the lies to God's truth and **choose to** believe the Lord's report
>
> ➤ Change your self-talk with truth (not just positive words)

The goal is to change what you say to yourself, choose to believe truth, and form different thoughts about your experiences and how you make sense of those experiences. Many times, you may not be aware of your self-talk or what you are thinking or believing. This chapter will help you **identify and challenge your thoughts**.

> If evil looked like evil, you would flee from it.
> If a lie looked like a lie, you would never believe it.

As you go through your inventory, you may find things that are interfering with your recovery or keeping you stuck. These are your "stuck points." Often your stuck points contribute to the "things you want to change" list from your heart check.

Create a page in your journal to use as a "Stuck Points" log.
You will add to this list as you work on your inventory and
pull from this list as you tackle your problematic thinking.

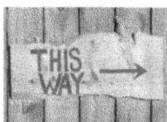
Stuck points may be conflicts between your beliefs before and after a traumatic experience. If you have experienced trauma that is keeping you stuck, tell your coach. Your coach will have additional resources to help you.

Discover and Overcome Stuck Points
First, Know What You Think

How Thought, Emotion, and Behavior Relate
Say the following situation occurs: Someone asks you to speak at an event in front of about 100 people. The situation triggers the thought, "I am going to mess this up." That thought leads to an emotion, and you experience nervousness. You then decline the opportunity to speak. The thought led to your emotion, which influenced the choice you made not to speak.

However, sometimes an emotion occurs without a thought to evoke the emotion. It may even seem unrelated to the current situation. Not all our thoughts are **conscious thoughts**, where we hear the words in our head. Beliefs stored in our **subconscious mind** may also trigger emotions. **Beliefs**, whether they are true or not true, are solid ideas that influence the way we see things for as long as we hold that belief. In the previous example, you may not think the words, "I am going to mess this up." But you may see yourself as a failure, and if so, this belief will make you nervous when speaking before a large group.

Discover Your Thoughts

To discover the thoughts behind the emotion, ask yourself why you have this emotion. What are you saying to yourself that causes these feelings? Is it the current situation or something outside of the situation that causes your mind to process this way?

To discover our thoughts and challenge and replace problematic thinking, we will use the "K.C.R." worksheets on the following pages.

Worksheet K – Know Your Thoughts

Use this worksheet to figure out what you are thinking or feeling in any given situation.

- If you are more aware of your feelings, fill in that column first. Then trace back the situation and discover the message you were saying to yourself.

- Use this worksheet as soon as you recognize a problem, so you are more likely to remember what you were saying to yourself. You may have more than one thought or emotion for a situation.

- Emotions are usually one-word answers. For example, "I feel sad" represents an emotion. "I feel like I can never do anything right." Is a thought or belief it is not an emotion.

A Situation Something Happens	B Thought/Belief What I tell myself	C Emotion What I feel

**Do not try to analyze if the thought is right or wrong;
simply identify what you are thinking.**

(Ask your coach for samples of completed worksheets and discuss your answers with your coach)

Worksheet C – Challenge Your thoughts

Now that you have identified what you think, challenge those thoughts. Are they the truth?
Answer all *relevant* questions below for each belief listed in column B on your "*K*" worksheet.

Situation *(Column A)*: _____

1. What was your part in this?

2. What part did other's play in the situation?

3. What are the facts of the situation? What new information, if any, has come to light?

Belief: _____ How much do you believe this thought? _____%

4. What other past experiences led to or supported this belief?

5. Does this belief fall into a problematic thinking pattern? _____ Explain.

6. Is your belief a habitual response, based in feelings, or based in facts?

7. What evidence supports this belief?   Is your source of information reliable?

8. What evidence suggests this belief is not true?

9. What assumptions were made?

10. Are you using words that are extreme/exaggerated (always, never, should, must, etc.)?

11. Are you taking a situation out of context, (focusing only on one aspect/irrelevant factors)?

12. Realistically, what are the chances your concerns will happen?

13. Are your interpretations accurate, or could you have misinterpreted the facts?

14. What does the bible say about you or the situation? Does it line up with your belief?

15. If your child, friend, or loved one came to you with your belief, what would you tell them?

Worksheet R – Replace Your Thoughts

After examining the situations and your beliefs in worksheet "C", you may begin to see some lies that you have believed. It is important to take everything you believe and hold it up to God's word. Does it line up with what the scripture says?

For instance:

❖ If shame is part of your beliefs, does it belong to you? Are you guilty? Blame goes to those with **responsibility and intent**. If something bad happened and you have some responsibility in it, yet you did not intend for it to happen, you should not carry guilt.

> *"Then Jesus said, 'Father, forgive them, for they do not know what they are doing.'" (Luke 23:34)*

> *"For the LORD sees not as man sees: man looks on the outward appearance, but the LORD looks on the heart." (1 Samuel 16:7)*

❖ If you are guilty of something, do you believe the lie that you are too bad for forgiveness? Do you believe that your mistakes define who you are? In Christ, when you take responsibility for your wrongs and repent *(turn away from it)* the Lord is faithful and just to forgive you. If you have remorse and turn away from wrongdoing, you no longer need to carry the weight of guilt.

> *"If we confess our sins, he is faithful and just to forgive us our sins and to cleanse us from all unrighteousness." (1 John 1:9)*

> *"For godly grief produces a repentance that leads to salvation without regret, whereas worldly grief produces death." (2 Corinthians 7:10)*

Consider the situation you wrote in the A column on your "K " worksheet.

• What is your true responsibility for the situation?

• What was the actual responsibility of others involved?

• Whom do you need to forgive? Do you need to forgive yourself?

• Do you need to seek forgiveness from the Lord, or make amends for past wrongs?

• What lies are you believing?

• How can you think differently about the situation?

• What is the truth? What can you say instead of the original thought/belief (from column B)?

• How strongly do you believe this new thought? _____%

• How much do you now believe the original thought? _____%

• Choose and memorize a verse that speaks about your problem or helps solidify the truth/new belief.

Chapter Seven

Self-control

Lesson 25 — Overwhelming Emotion

Sometimes life happens too quickly, emotions are too strong, anger is too overwhelming, or the fear is too great, for us to analyze a situation. When a moment of life becomes this overpowering, it is difficult to function or even pray.

Anger and fear are two damaging emotions when they are misunderstood, and they can keep us trapped in a deep web of false beliefs, sometimes leading us to fear or blame God. These emotions can drive us to a place where we cannot pray and seek the Lord, giving the enemy free rein. Then he can speak any lie he wants into our ears. One thought feeds another, until the situation seems utterly hopeless. Have you ever been there?

This chapter will introduce different biblical strategies for self-control—strategies that can stop your mind from spinning before you lose control. These are "in the moment" tools. If you learned other **healthy strategies** for handling emotions that work for you, continue to use them. However, many times our coping mechanisms **are not healthy**. Consider the impact of your coping skills.

Questions to Ponder

25.1) How often do you lose control of your thoughts or actions when experiencing anger?

25.2) How often do you lose control of your thoughts or actions when experiencing fear or an unknown situation?

25.3) Write about a recent situation in which you felt your emotions spin you out of control.

25.4) Thinking back, can you identify what first triggered the emotion (what started it)?

Self-control is a fruit of the Spirit. The ability to control yourself is only possible with the Lord. Your heart can change, but you cannot change it. In our flesh we can control behavior temporarily, but only the Spirit of God can change the corruption in our heart that drives our behavior. We cannot change our sin nature any more than a leopard can change his spots.

For I do not understand my own actions. For I do not do what I want, but I do the very thing I hate. (Romans 7:15)

Can the Ethiopian change his skin, or the leopard his spots? Neither are you able to do good—you who are accustomed to doing evil. (Jeremiah 13:23, BSB)

Questions to Ponder

25.5) What are some healthy ways you cope with difficult emotions?

25.6) What are some detrimental ways you cope with difficult emotions?

25.7) How have poor coping skills harmed you and those around you?

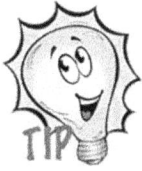

Emotions can become your prison.
Self-control is freedom *not* to respond instead of giving your emotions control.

It is freedom **NOT** to act in anger.

It is freedom **NOT** to stay home out of fear.

It is **NOT** legalism; it is **NOT** a prison.

Emotions: Are They Good or Bad?

God created us in His image, and He has emotions. He gets angry, He loves, and He grieves. Jesus wept at the death of Lazarus and turned over tables in the temple when there was injustice in His Father's house. It is not a sin to have emotions; it is sin if we act on those emotions in a wrong way.

For we do not have a high priest who is unable to sympathize with our weaknesses, but one who in every respect has been tempted as we are, yet without sin.
(Hebrews 4:15)

Many people find emotional regulation extremely difficult. Even the most emotionally stable people have moments where emotions dictate their actions. Unlike us, God deals well with His emotions. He is always just and good regardless of His feelings.

The anger of man does not produce the and kill and righteousness of God.
(Ephesians 4:26)

Emotions are beneficial in that they give us information. Anger alerts us to injustice; fear alerts us to danger; grief and pain teach compassion; love teaches us about the Lord.

In our sin nature, we misuse our emotions. Fear may compel us to control and use people, to manipulate circumstances, or to protect ourselves from perceived dangers aroused by our jealousy or insecurity. Pride and selfishness may stir anger when we do not like the circumstance or how people behave or respond. Anger leads to hate, gossip, slander, and other forms of sin.

We have an enemy whispering in our ears. His main tactic for destruction involves our thoughts and emotions. He feeds on our fears and insecurities, telling lies that make a normal situation seem like something it is not. Jesus came to overcome the enemy and the power of sin and death in us. The enemy tries to use our emotions against us, **hoping we will reject the abundant life Christ wants us to possess**. When we understand our emotions, **they can alert us to and stop the plans of the enemy**. The more we understand why we feel as we do, the more we can spot deception and false thinking.

The thief comes only to steal destroy. I came that they may have life and have it abundantly. (John 10:10)

Emotional Control

Do not allow your emotions to draw you into sin, fear, or anger. Do not allow them to continue unabated without understanding or resolution. Recognize and accept your emotions. If you fear or reject your feelings, you may bury them. Suppressed emotion causes anxiety and other mental health issues. It is important to acknowledge emotion, **but if you do not control the emotion, it will control you**.

Be angry and do not sin; do not let the sun go down on your anger.
(James 1:20)

For God gave us a spirit not of fear but of power and love and self-control.
(2 Timothy 1:7)

Questions to Ponder

25.8) Question your feelings. What is the most prevalent emotion you experience?

25.9) Do you shut down emotion?

25.10) Do your emotional responses come long after the situation?

25.11) Are you an emotional person? Do your emotions control your decision-making process?

How Behavior Works

To break the chains of codependency, anger, mental illness, addiction, and so on, we must **literally break a chain**. A situation, circumstance, or physical sensation triggers a **thought**, and that thought triggers a **feeling/emotion**, which triggers a **behavior/action**, which triggers a **consequence**. The consequence often triggers another thought, which triggers another emotion, which triggers another behavior and another consequence. The cycle continues, tightening our emotional shackles and leading us into a deep, tangled web of confusion.

Detrimental thoughts are the start of that chain. It is best to take those thoughts captive at the chain's beginning. The more you allow thoughts to go unchecked, the longer your chain and the more links you must destroy to release yourself from your chain. The book of James illustrates this process:

But each person is tempted [thoughts] when he is lured and enticed by his own
desire [emotions]. Then desire when it has conceived gives birth to sin [behavior]
and sin when it is fully grown brings forth death [consequence].
(James 1: 14 – 15)

Question to Ponder

25.12) Write about a time when you experienced this process play out in your own life.

Trust and Humility

The best weapon against overwhelming emotions is to humble yourself and trust in the Lord. Do not assume you know the answers or that the world has your answers. You may have part of it right, and the world may have part of it right. God, who created everything, is the only one with the big picture and all the answers. God cares for you. Leaning on His truth will bring you peace and healing.

> *Trust in the LORD with all your heart, and do not lean on your own understanding. In all your ways acknowledge him, and he will make straight your paths. Be not wise in your own eyes; fear the LORD, and turn away from evil. It will be healing to your flesh and refreshment to your bones. (Proverbs 3:5 – 8)*

> *Blessed be the God and Father of our Lord Jesus Christ, the Father of mercies and God of all comfort, who comforts us in all our affliction, so that we may be able to comfort those who are in any affliction, with the comfort with which we ourselves are comforted by God. For as we share abundantly in Christ's sufferings, so through Christ we share abundantly in comfort too. (2 Corinthians 1:3 – 5)*

Questions to Ponder

25.13) Do you believe God cares about you and cares for you?

25.14) What are some ways that the Lord has taken care of you in the past?

Lesson 26 — Coping Strategies

How Should We Deal with Emotion?

Scripture shows us the correct way to deal with emotions in first Peter:

> *__Humble yourselves__, therefore, under the mighty hand of God so that at the proper time he may exalt you, __casting all your anxieties on him__, because he cares for you. __Be sober-minded; be watchful__. Your adversary the devil prowls around like a roaring lion, seeking someone to devour. __Resist him, firm in your faith__, knowing that the __same kinds of suffering are being experienced by your brotherhood__ throughout the world. And __after you have suffered a little while__, the God of all grace, who has called you to his eternal glory in Christ, __will himself restore, confirm, strengthen, and establish you__.*
> *(1 Peter 5:6 – 10)*

Let emotions alert you to a situation and give you information:

➤ **Humble yourself**. Do not rely on your way of thinking to understand. Seek God's wisdom and give your concerns about the situation to Him. Tell Him how you feel! He cares for you, and He will help you.

➤ **Keep your mind sober.** Do not use alcohol or drugs to run away from your emotions. *(Note: This is referring to self-medicating. Never stop taking medications prescribed under a qualified physician's care without your doctor's guidance. This may cause serious harm.)*

  ○ A sober mind Is also a steady, sound mind. Do not allow your thoughts to spin out of control. Take them to the Lord first.

➤ **Keep guard against the lies of the enemy.** He will try to spin you up or use your emotions against you. Do not let him.

➤ **Resist the enemy:**

  ○ Trust that the Lord will keep you in whatever you are going through.

  ○ Know you are not alone in your pain; God is with you, and others have suffered what you are suffering and come through it.

  ○ Understand that your suffering is only for a short time. When the season is over, God Himself will restore, confirm, strengthen, and establish you.

  ○ Seek and believe truth.

The following strategies are the first steps in managing your emotions.
The moment you feel negative emotions or face temptation,
S.T.O.P. then **T.H.I.N.K.**

Questions to Ponder

Read the following two strategies, (STOP and THINK) and put them into practice.

26.1) Write about using the strategies.

26.2) How did the strategies help you?

26.3) Where did you find the strategies difficult to implement?

To remember the ways in which the Lord has blessed you, cared for you, and comforted you, is like a memorial to God commemorating all He has done in your life.

Create/Use a praise journal.

Every day, write the ways you can give thanks to the Lord in your journal!

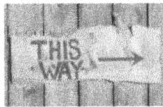

Share your Praise Journal with your coach.
Read your journal when you have times of doubt.

Strategy: S.T.O.P.

The acrostic S.T.O.P. can help you remember what to do when a strong emotion comes as a surprise. It is important **to stop at the initial thought** *before the emotions are get too powerful and spin you out of control.*

Treat your emotions like a stop sign. You are not trying to stop the emotion; you are stopping your thinking. When an emotion surprises you or appears negative, recognize it as you would a stop sign when you are driving. The vehicle of thought must come to a complete stop! When thoughts spin up, it is exceedingly difficult to regain control.

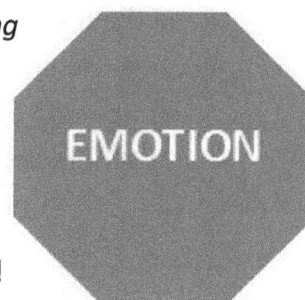

EMOTION

Stay

Stay at the feet of Jesus. Become grounded in the present. Do not hang out in the past or look toward future concerns. Focus on the here and now. Find a point of focus, like the chair you are sitting on, for example. The only thing required of you is simply to breathe. Put your concerns on a shelf in your mind. Wait until you are in a better place or the Lord directs you to act before taking the concern off your shelf.

They who wait for the LORD shall renew their strength; they shall mount up with wings like eagles; they shall run and not be weary; they shall walk and not faint. (Isaiah 40:31)

Trust

Trust that God has it. This is the power of letting. **Let** God hear your emotion, **let** Him know your concern, your anger, or your fear, and **let** Him take responsibility for the outcome. In things out of your control, do not search for ways to force the situation into your control. Remember, the Lord knows what is best, and He sees the situation clearer than you do.

Trust in the LORD with all your heart, and do not lean on your own understanding.
In all your ways acknowledge him, and he will make straight your paths. (Proverbs 3:5 – 6)

Observe

Observe the conditions that could contribute to the emotion. Are you tired? Hungry? Sick? Overwhelmed? Did you take medicine? Ladies, are you near your cycle? All these things can magnify the emotion you feel. Examine the situation. What is happening that you dislike? What is concerning you? Is the emotion you are experiencing out of proportion to the circumstance?

But if we judged ourselves truly, we would not be judged. (2 Corinthians 11:31)

Pray

Pray that the Lord will reveal what you need to know or the actions you should take. Be humble and do not lean on your own understanding. Remain calm: Time is on your side. Wait for an answer from the Lord.

If any of you lacks wisdom, let him ask God, who gives generously to all
without reproach, and it will be given him. (James 1:5)

Strategy: T.H.I.N.K.

First use the STOP strategy, then you can THINK.

Turn

Turn the emotion into information. What information does the emotion tell you? What are your actual beliefs about yourself or your situation? Seek the Lord for the truth about the situation.

> *But I say, walk by the Spirit, and you will not gratify the desires of the flesh. (Galatians 5:16)*

Honest

Be honest and humble. What are you learning about yourself from the emotion? Are you being inconsiderate or self-centered? Are you insecure or worried? Are your expectations reasonable?

> *If we say we have no sin, we deceive ourselves, and the truth is not in us. (1 John 1:8)*

Investigate

Investigate all the options. Identify your assumptions and look for alternative plausible explanations. What information is still unknown? Are the expectations of others reasonable? How could the enemy be using your emotion to cause harm? What lies are you hearing or trusting?

> *The simple believes everything, but the prudent gives thought to his steps. (Proverbs 14:15)*

No

No snap decisions. Learn to tell yourself no. Step back and take time to assess the situation. Gather your thoughts, ask questions, and get truthful information. Powerful emotions tempt us to jump to conclusions. You cannot take back a snap response, and it often will do more damage than good. Before you act, give yourself a cooling-off period to process your emotions and what happened to trigger them. Allow God time to move on your behalf in the situation. Avoiding impulsiveness prevents choices we regret. **The path of least regret is rarely the easy or quick path.**

> *If one gives an answer before he hears, it is his folly and shame. (Proverbs 18:13)*

Keep

Keep sober-minded to prepare your mind for action. Guard your mind by focusing your thoughts on the Kingdom of God and whatever is true, honorable, just, pure, lovely, commendable, excellent, and anything worthy of praise (see Philippians 4:8).

> *Therefore, preparing your minds for action, and being sober-minded, set your hope fully on the grace that will be brought to you at the revelation of Jesus Christ. (1 Peter 1:13)*

Chapter Eight

Perseverance

Lesson 27 — Persevere

What is perseverance? The Scripture uses words like "steadfastness," "endurance," and "patience." The Merriam-Webster dictionary says perseverance is persistence in doing something despite difficulty or delay in achieving success. It is hard to keep doing the right things, to keep having faith, when the answers seem far away. It is hard to keep on when the battle seems endless, and to keep standing up in our weakness. Yet we prosper if we do not give up.

And let us not grow weary of doing good, for in due season we will reap,
if we do not give up. (Galatians 6:9)

We Must Persevere

The Lord allows us to experience trials to test us and strengthen our character. We enter the Kingdom of God through many tribulations. (Tribulation: A cause or state of great trouble or suffering.)

In the world you will have tribulation. But take heart; I have overcome the world.
(John 16:33)

When you do something new, prepare a new product, or promote a new program, you test it, right? You will run trials to check what works and remove any bugs. Tests and trials are also a necessary part of the process of transformation to make us a new creation in Christ.

Perseverance through Difficulty Is the Growing Pains of Character

The Lord knows the hidden things in our heart that we struggle to see. We may think we have overcome a character defect, but when the right trial comes along, that defect can rise to the surface again. Our trials and stresses shed light on our weaknesses, helping us to see where we are and how much we have grown. Each trial we face brings us deeper into the root of our character defects so God can do a complete work in our hearts.

The Lord does not allow trials and tests so He can grade our progress. Our trials benefit us, helping us see where we need to grow and how far we have come, refining us, making us perfect and complete. They strengthen our faith, nurture our love, make our hope certain, and mold us into a reflection of Jesus—the person God predestined us to become to receive His eternal promise.

More than that, we rejoice in our sufferings, knowing that suffering produces endurance, and
endurance produces character, and character produces hope, and hope does not put us to
shame, because God's love has been poured into our hearts through the Holy Spirit who has
been given to us. (Romans 5:3 – 5)

For you know that the testing of your faith produces steadfastness. And let steadfastness have
its full effect, that you may be perfect and complete, lacking in nothing. (James 1:3 – 4)

For those whom he foreknew he also predestined <u>to be conformed to the image of his Son</u>, in
order that he might be the firstborn among many brothers. (Romans 8:29)

When we persevere, we are blessed with eternal victory!

And you will be hated by all for my name's sake.
But the one who endures to the end will be saved. (Matthew 10:22)

Be the Tree!

Blessed is the man who <u>trusts in the LORD</u>, whose <u>trust is the LORD</u>. He is like a tree
planted by water, that sends out its roots by the stream, and does not fear when heat
comes, for its leaves remain green, and is not anxious in the year of drought, for it does
not cease to bear fruit. (Jeremiah 17:7 – 8)

He is like a tree planted by streams of water that yields its fruit in its season, and
its leaf does not wither. In all that he does, he prospers. (Psalm 1:1 – 3)

Perseverance starts with trust. God is the only place worthy of your trust. We trust in Him, but **He IS also our trust**. If you have a dozen eggs, you can put some eggs in a basket and others in your refrigerator, in a pan, on your counter, and even save a couple to throw at someone's house. It is the same with trust. You can put trust in the Lord and put trust in your shelter, in weapons, in your skill, in your wisdom, in your family, or in your friends. Jeremiah is telling us to trust in the Lord, but also to make the Lord the place which holds all our trust. Our trust **is** the Lord, **like putting all your eggs in one basket; you put all you have in Him.**

Scripture compares perseverance to a tree planted by water. The tree planted can stand in the heat; it does not wither from drought; instead, it always produces fruit. The tree's roots keep it connected to the source of life-giving water. **The Lord is our source of life.** When we stay connected to our source, we can stand the heat of the refiner's fire and will not wither in times of lack. Our lives will never stop bearing fruit. We will prosper in all we do because we stay grounded in our source.

And he is before all things, and in him all things hold together. (Colossians 1:17)

Stay Grounded in Your Source

You cast off many things during your inventory, emptying yourself of past pain, lies, fear, sin, and guilt. Now it is time to put on something new. You must replace what you took off, filling the holes left in your heart. The trick is to fill them with suitable things.

First, you put off your old self and renewed your mind in truth. This was your inventory and heart check. It is plausible that you will discover more things to put off as you walk through life with God. The process of removing lies and renewing your mind is ongoing. After putting off your old self, you must put on your new self in Christ. The book of Romans tells us the **first thing** you put on is Jesus, so you can be transformed into His likeness.

To put off your old self, which belongs to your former manner of life and is corrupt through deceitful
desires, and to be renewed in the spirit of your minds, and to put on the new self, created after the
likeness of God in true righteousness and holiness. (Ephesians 4:22 – 24)

But put on the Lord Jesus Christ, and make no provision for the flesh, to gratify its desires.
(Romans 13:14)

Jesus is our source. Once we put Him on, we stand strong by putting on the whole armor of God. **This is how we become the tree planted by the water.**

Put on the whole armor of God, that you may be able to stand
against the schemes of the devil. (Ephesians 6:11)

Read Ephesians 6:11 – 18

This armor, mentioned in Ephesians, is our relationship with God. The **belt of truth** keeps the armor on. Rebuking the enemy's lies in exchange for God's truth, knowing His word, and living a life of honesty and integrity, keeps the other pieces of armor in place. The **breastplate of righteousness** protects your heart, keeping your heart in check so no sin can creep in and take hold. Your **shoes** guard your walk. Walk in the footsteps of Jesus in every moment of your day. The **gospel of peace** keeps you confident. In every circumstance, keep your **shield of faith**—your trust in God. Every dart the enemy can throw will bounce off this shield. Guard your mind with the **helmet of salvation**. The enemy attacks your mind, the place which births emotion, desire, sin, doubt, love, and hate. When you think wrongly, the enemy gains a foothold, and everything goes wrong. Rest assured, you are the Lord's, and His Word is true for you.

Your offensive tool is the **sword of the Spirit**, fighting against enemy's attacks. The Holy Spirit deciphers God's Word, speaking directly into your life. Finally, **cover everything in prayer** and pray for your brothers and sisters in Christ.

When you dress in God's armor, you can stand!

Questions to Ponder
Read the following CHOICE strategy and put it into practice.

27.1) Write about using the strategy.

27.2) How did the strategy help you?

27.3) Where did you find the strategy difficult to implement?

Strategy: C.H.O.I.C.E.

You will stand strong with the Lord each day when you choose well. **Choose** Him first in each moment, and you will persevere every day, in everything.

Character

Choose excellent character in trial. STOP and THINK so you do not react in your flesh, but in the wisdom and love of the Lord.

> *But the one who looks into the perfect law, the law of liberty, and perseveres, being no hearer who forgets but a doer who acts, he will be blessed in his doing. (James 1:25)*

Hope

Place your hope in the Lord. Remember the promises of God and count on them.

> *Rejoice in hope, be patient in tribulation, be constant in prayer. (Romans 12:12)*

Optimism

Optimism in trials brings us joy, because we are confident that the Lord will work through everything for our benefit. Keep a heart of gratitude, remembering the Lord's provisions. Know with certainty that He finishes the work He starts. Optimism comes from hope. Hope deferred makes the heart sick.

> *Count it all joy, my brothers, when you meet trials of various kinds, for you know that the testing of your faith produces steadfastness. And let steadfastness have its full effect, that you may be perfect and complete, lacking in nothing. (James 1:2 – 4)*

Immovable

Be the immovable tree. Stand firm and do not allow your faith to waiver. The Lord has your back. He is the strength and the source allowing you to stand.

> *Therefore, my beloved brothers, be steadfast, immovable, always abounding in the work of the Lord, knowing that in the Lord your labor is not in vain. (1 Corinthians 15:58)*

Connected

Stay connected to your source. Keep the Word of the Lord in you and live your life in Him. Allow everything you do and all that you are to come from Him.

> *If you abide in me, and my words abide in you, ask whatever you wish, and it will be done for you. (John 15:7)*

Escape

Escape from flesh temptations. The Lord provides a way to escape temptation, including temptations to doubt God, fear circumstances, act in anger, or gratify a desire contrary to the Lord.

> *No temptation has overtaken you that is not common to man. God is faithful, and he will not let you be tempted beyond your ability, but with the temptation he will also provide the way of escape, that you may be able to endure it. (1 Corinthians 10:13)*

Chapter Nine

Anger Management

Lesson 28 — Dealing with Anger

Why Do We Get Angry?

Many circumstances trigger anger. Anger may **result from an injustice** perpetrated against us or another we love. **Or it can be motivated by a desire not to feel guilt or shame.** To **avoid looking** at our own sins, mistakes, or flaws, we may shift the blame to other people or circumstances, projecting our anger onto the victim of our wrongs.

Anger is a way our mind protects us from feeling another emotion, such as fear or pain. The adrenaline rush that comes with anger covers up disturbing feelings and **provides a sense of invulnerability**, which allows us to escape upsetting emotions in the moment. This anger is a **secondary emotion**, and to deal with it, we must first expose the emotion that triggered it.

Remember the acrostic **H.U.F.F.** to discover what is hiding beneath your anger:

- **H**urt – Physical or emotional pain, accusations, guilt, shame, feeling disregarded, unimportant, devalued, rejected, or unlovable.

- **U**nfairness – Unfair circumstances, not getting your way, envy (someone else has what you want), or believing nothing is fair in life.

- **F**ear – Feeling powerless, anxious, worried, intimidated, jealous, fearful of loss or the future, or other frightening circumstances.

- **F**rustration – Consistent mistakes, failure, circumstances not working out the way you want, hopelessness, disappointment, helplessness, feeling out of control, feeling life is too difficult, or experiencing many minor irritations and daily hassles.

In anger, when a person offends or hurts you, you may retaliate by returning the same hurt. For example, if a person belittles or rejects you, you may find something for which to ridicule or reject them. You are no longer the one demeaned; they are. A person who feels powerless or insecure may act out in a fit of rage to feel empowered and safe. Anger responses push your burden onto another while giving you a false sense of control. Your burden still exists beneath the mask of rage, but now it has become another's burden as well.

Anger begets more anger. Those receiving your anger often retaliate in anger. They feel threatened, responding with their own defensive actions, and escalating the conflict. Sometimes, however, people may flee your wrath, responding with hurt and fear instead of lashing out. They may distance themselves from you to escape your anger.

Defining Anger and Aggression

Anger can range from mild irritation to fierce rage and may lead to aggression. It is important to catch your anger right away before it escalates. **Aggression is deliberate harm to another,** physical or otherwise. Common aggressive behaviors include violence, breaking things, yelling, and screaming, but aggression may also appear passive.

Passive aggression is manipulation, which manifests as seeking revenge, sarcasm, ridicule, shunning, or slander. People often display passive aggressive behaviors with bitterness and resentment. They may respond by refusing, delaying, or being inefficient in doing something with the intent to cause another harm or "get them back." An example of passive aggressive behavior is refusing to do a task until the one who benefits from the task does something you want first. Passive aggressive people do not discuss their concerns. They may rationalize their behavior as "fairness" or deny their anger altogether.

Righteous Anger

We may become angry when people hurt us through no fault of our own, or when we see an injustice that goes unpunished. People disrespect the God we love, the innocent get hurt , and evil prevails. What angers the Lord can and should anger us. While we may justify this anger, when we respond to it with bitterness, resentment, and hate, we are sinning in our anger. To react in anger makes a situation worse, preventing others from understanding our feelings or resolving the issue. Whether it is selfish or righteous, we must not sin in our anger.

> *Be angry and do not sin; do not let the sun go down on your anger,*
> *and give no opportunity to the devil. (Ephesians 4:26 – 27)*

It may seem like ignoring or avoiding anger keeps peace. The reality is that avoiding a problem allows anger to fester inside. As you stew on the situation, you give the enemy the opportunity to plant thoughts and schemes, amplifying the conflict in your mind and tempting you to act in a way that escalates the situation. Not letting the sun go down on your anger means you should deal with your feelings right away. This prevents escalation or avoidance, which aggravates the situation. The longer you hold on to anger, the more opportunity you give the devil to manipulate it.

Anger Misconceptions

One common misconception about anger is that people believe they just need to vent, and everything will be better. It is not good to suppress or ignore your anger, but it is just as harmful to vent your anger or unleash your rage on another. Not only do you crush another's spirit, but **every time you lash out, it reinforces your aggressive behavior**. You form a belief that you must act out or the anger will consume you. When we frequently reinforce detrimental anger responses, they become automatic. Anger becomes our "go-to" for dealing with any situation we dislike. **Anger becomes a habit.**

Anger is not hereditary, but witnessing extreme anger responses as a child can cause it to become a habitual response for you. You may be unaware of the force behind the anger driving your behavior. If this is true of you, attempt to realize the moment you feel hostility and take your anger captive. Healthy handling of anger prevents it from festering like a neglected wound, releasing the anger in a way that resolves the problem.

False Invulnerability

Another misconception about anger is believing your intimidation and aggression make people respect you or treat you well. You may feel that being enraged makes people listen or give you what you want or need. The truth is that, while angry reactions may cause people to fear you, pretend to like you, or guard their words around you, **they do not respect you for your anger**. Almost everyone responds better when treated kindly. Even if a person is compliant, angry bullying breeds resentment.

Uncontrollable Anger

It is a lie that you cannot help how you respond or control yourself when angry. Anger is not destructive behavior, nor does it cause aggression. The intensity of the emotion makes it seem beyond your ability to control, but anger is like any other emotion. Despite how it feels, anger is only a signal giving you information that alerts you to a problem. You can **choose to control** how you express anger and handle it in a way that does not cause physical or emotional abuse.

Verbal or physical aggression, damaging property, or hurting people is not anger. These are behaviors resulting from anger when we do not manage the emotion in a healthy, biblical way.

You must separate anger from behaviors, recognizing that they are distinct from one another. You cannot prevent anger, but **you can choose and control how you respond to that anger.** This realization empowers you to stop your anger from escalating or festering.

> **Recognize** anger at the first sign of wrong thinking, before it overwhelms you.
> **Choose** to deal with the emotions behind the anger.
> **Choose** to resolve issues instead of allowing anger to fester.

Deal with Your Anger

If you struggle with anger or it seems out of control, pay close attention to what triggered the anger. When did you first feel irritation? Are you responding without thinking or out of habit? Is your feeling based on wrong thinking or truth? What is the emotion or stronghold (the influencing belief) behind the anger? What triggered your anger? Is your anger justified? How can you resolve this situation?

How Angry Are You?

Consider your anger like a ladder with ten rungs. The ground represents complete calm with no irritation or resentment. At the first sign of irritation or annoyance, you climbed to the bottom rung of your ladder. The top rung of the ladder represents explosive anger that causes aggressive actions. Where are you on your anger ladder? The higher on your ladder, the more unstable you are. Your goal is to keep your feet on solid ground. The best time to get control is on the bottom rung.

Watch for physical signs of anger. If you have trouble identifying anger until you are way up on your anger ladder, watch for physical changes in your body that may indicate you are angry, such as a rapid heartbeat, faster breathing, tension in your body (i.e., clenched hands or jaw), restlessness, pacing, shaking your leg, tapping of feet or hands, sweating, or trembling.

> <u>Questions to Ponder</u>
> Keep track of your anger this week. Answer the questions about your anger experiences:
> 28.1) **What physical symptoms accompany your anger? Where are you on your anger ladder when you notice these symptoms?**
> 28.2) **What experiences or circumstances triggered your anger?**
> 28.3) **Use the following calming strategies this week. Which works best for you?**

Keep Calm: Fast-acting strategies to use in the heat of the moment

Respond, don't react

Take a timeout. This strategy involves stepping away until you can handle the situation well. Leave, if possible, or stop the discussion until a later time. Stop, relax, and think so you can respond well instead of reacting in anger.

Preempt your anger. Prepare ahead of time if there is a likelihood that addressing a conflict may end with one or both people involved losing control of their anger. Agree, before emotions get out of control, that either person may call a time-out to pause the conversation and finish the discussion later. This gives both people time to deal with anger, preventing escalation.

Relax and breathe

The fastest way to calm down is to **focus on your breathing**. Deep breathing from your diaphragm causes a physical change, which calms your body and mind. Be aware that chest breathing does not work. You need to inhale from the deepest part of your gut and visualize all the stress leaving your body as you exhale. Exhale slowly, for longer than the inhale. If it helps, imagine a peaceful place while breathing.

Exercise — Push a wall

Physical exertion relieves tension in your body. Clean your house, go for a walk, or lift weights at the gym. Anger causes energy, and getting that energy out of your body clears your mind to deal with the anger. **Do not hit** a pillow or punching bag, as this may have the opposite effect. A fight response is created in your mind when you hit objects, feeding your body with even more energy.

One effective method for releasing the energy from anger is to push a wall. Walk up to a **sturdy** wall or doorframe. Do not run, as you may push right through it! Place your hands on the wall and your feet away from it, as if you are trying to push the wall down. Push as hard as you can; yell at the wall if you want. The goal is to push on the wall until your arms and legs grow weak and you physically cannot push any more. Release all the angry energy from your body onto the wall. Then you will have the ability to process what angered you and how to handle the situation.

Healthy Processing of Anger

Anger makes it difficult to keep from saying or doing the wrong thing, so in a moment of anger, stop and be **SILENT**. Once you have calmed down, you can process what you are feeling.

Use the S.I.L.E.N.T strategy that follows to help process anger and avoid aggressive behaviors

> ## Questions to Ponder
> Read the following S.I.L.E.N.T. strategy and put it into practice.
>
> **28.4) Write about using the strategy.**
>
> **28.5) How did the strategy help you?**
>
> **28.6) Where did you find the strategy difficult to implement?**

Strategy: S.I.L.E.N.T.

Stop

Catching anger right away is the key to managing it. Identify it, then take steps to clear your mind. Look for the physical signs of anger. When you first notice anger, take a time-out to walk, exercise, practice breathing or relaxation techniques, or talk with your coach or accountability partner.

Identify

Identify the cues or events that cause your hostility. Is the neighbor leaving trash in your yard or playing music too loud? Were you on hold too long, or did another's incompetence cause you to fail? Is someone stealing from you, or degrading you and spreading lies? What is the triggering event? What warning signs alert you to anger?

Look for the **physical cues** (i.e., bodily responses such as tight jaw or muscles, fast heart rate, surge of adrenalin, etc.), **behavioral cues** (glaring, raising your voice, etc.), **emotional cues** (other feelings like fear, hurt, jealousy, etc. that accompany or precede your anger), and **thought cues** (any thoughts that are increasing your hostility. Ask: Do I see images of aggression or have ideas of revenge?).

Ladder

Remember the anger ladder. Monitor your anger. If you struggle with severe anger issues, check your place on the anger ladder each morning and throughout the day. Write about it in your journal. Manage your anger on a moment-by-moment basis. Examine your cues and the related event and note the highest rung you climbed on the anger ladder. How are you bringing your feet back to ground level?

Explore

Explore the feelings and situations behind the anger. After you have identified the specific conflict, try to go further. What information can you learn from your anger? What about this situation caused you anger? Is a relationship unhealthy? Are you being mistreated, manipulated, or abused? Are you feeling inadequate or afraid of something? Do you want what you cannot have? How does this situation impact your life?

Negotiate

Negotiate the solution. Are you offended because of past experiences or assumptions? Is the perceived wrong legitimate? Are you being reasonable or taking something personally? What was your intent? Is it possible the other person did not intend harm or had a good motive? Should you resolve the conflict or deal with it in your heart? Discuss the issue with the person involved in love.

Take

Take back your rights. You can resolve a conflict without allowing people to walk all over you. You have a legitimate right to be treated with respect and dignity. Conflict resolution always involves forgiving, but that does not mean you must put yourself in a position to continue suffering harm from another. Be assertive but not aggressive when standing up for yourself.

Chapter Ten

Anxiety & Fear Management

Lesson 29 — Anxiety

Everyone experiences fear—it is a normal emotion. Fear comes in many forms, including anxiety, jealousy, nervousness, insecurity, pride, or a strong, terrified response of panic. Like every other emotion, **fear gives you information**, alerting you to emotional or physical danger. If you listen to the information your fear provides, you will learn to navigate tough situations and avoid harmful situations.

Anxiety usually results from stress or worry—fear about what is happening or going to happen. Stress is normal and can occur in pleasant or unpleasant situations. It is normal to have some anxiety when preparing to give a speech, perform, or confront a difficult situation. Anxiety alerts you to the possibility of failure and urges caution. It tells you a situation is important and requires extra attention, or to prepare for a potentially negative response. Normal anxiety occurs in a known situation, circumstance, or environment, and it leaves when the stressor is no longer present.

Anxiety manifests in physical symptoms such as a clenched jaw, tight muscles in the neck and back, headaches, chest pain, rapid heartbeat, or shortness of breath. It can cause a physical sense of dread, often described as a knot in the pit of the stomach. Anxiety makes it difficult to concentrate; it causes you to spin up, becoming restless and "on edge."

> Because anxiety includes such an intense physical component, managing your physical symptoms first can help your mind process the thoughts causing your anxiety.

Problematic Anxiety

Anxiety that exists when there is no threat or danger and interferes with daily life may be the sign of an anxiety disorder. This form of anxiety is a response to a stressor that exists only in our thoughts. Sometimes we are not even aware of the thoughts or beliefs that trigger the anxiety.

Problematic anxiety is unsubstantiated, constant worry. It may cause you to avoid situations, fearing failure or the reactions of others. It may cause panic attacks seemingly without reason. Or it can manifest as an irrational fear or avoidance of a person, object, place, or situation that carries little or no threat of danger. Anxiety creates a need for control. One way an anxious mind tries to grasp control is with obsessive behaviors, such as Obsessive-Compulsive Disorder (OCD). Obsessive behaviors may include constant checking of things or excessive touching, arranging, or cleaning.

Anxiety creates anxiety. For someone with an anxiety disorder, just the prospect of having stress or experiencing a panic attack can cause or increase anxiety. People often cause themselves anxiety by inventing self-defeating beliefs to escape their sense of dread.

Questions to Ponder

29.1) How do fear and anxiety affect your life?

29.2) Do you experience fear of social situations or other situations in which most people do not experience fear?

Anxiety without a Cause

Does it seem your anxiety has no origin or cause? This can happen with a **substance-induced anxiety disorder**, which occurs when anxiety symptoms develop from taking or stopping a drug. Alcohol, stimulants, caffeine, and some medications can cause an imbalance in the brain, which results in anxiety. Symptoms often cease within several weeks after the person stops using the substance.

Anxiety that originates from substance abuse affects a person's normal ability to cope with stressors, both new and old. Connecting substance-induced anxiety to past trauma can cause the symptoms to persist, even after the person ceases using the substance. If, however, anxiety was present before the use of a substance, it is not "substance-induced."

Suppressed emotions are another possible, hidden cause of anxiety. Many people cut off from their feelings because experiences have taught them that expressing emotion is wrong or even dangerous. People raised in an environment that did not allow them to understand or express their emotion often struggle with suppressed emotions.

Like anger, **anxiety is a common secondary emotion**; it is the emotion experienced instead of the suppressed emotion. If you cannot identify the situation that is making you anxious, it is possible there is an underlying emotion behind your anxiety. Many people who were raised without understanding emotions consider emotions weakness and reject them. People who do not express emotions well may experience anxiety in place of difficult emotions. The solution is learning to acknowledge and express your feelings and discover why you do not feel safe expressing the emotion.

Questions to Ponder

29.3) Do you experience anxiety resulting from taking, starting, or stopping an illegal drug, medication, or alcohol?

29.4) Are you able to express emotions such as grief, anger, pain, or sadness?

29.5) When do you consider it inappropriate to show emotions? When do you hide them?

29.6) If you struggle to express emotion, do you know why?

Fear leads us to want control, to protect ourselves. With anxiety, we try to control circumstances and situations around us, but in fact, **we can only control our own actions**.

The antidote to fear is trust in God, knowing yourself and God, and receiving His perfect love.

There is no fear in love, but perfect love casts out fear. For fear has to do with punishment, and whoever fears has not been perfected in love. (1 John 4:18)

When I am afraid, I put my trust in you. (Psalm 56:3)

Questions to Ponder

29.7) What situations are you still trying to control?

29.8) What is the fear behind your desire to control those situations?

29.9) Does your attempt at control alleviate the fear?

29.10) What different response to fear could you try that may lead to a better outcome?

Lesson 30 – Combat Anxiety & Panic Attacks

Anxiety disorders are a never-ending circle. Anxious thoughts lead to physical symptoms, which lead to behaviors that maintain and increase the anxiety.

It starts with a thought or belief. Sometimes we experience the symptoms of anxiety first and are unaware of the thought or belief causing it. As a result, we assume our thoughts come from experiencing the emotion, but the truth is that the physical sensations we feel come from our thoughts.

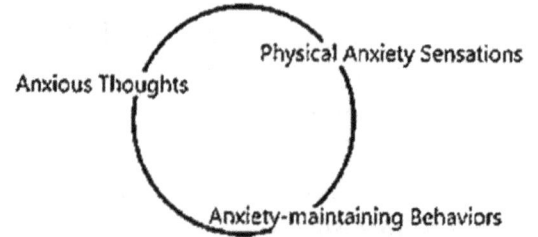

Anxious Thoughts — Physical Anxiety Sensations — Anxiety-maintaining Behaviors

We choose behaviors we expect will improve our anxiety, such as isolating from social scenes, attempting to take control, or avoiding challenging situations. These behaviors **lead to new beliefs**: We assume we are incapable or out of control. The new beliefs maintain or even increase the anxiety, and then this cycle repeats.

To break the cycle, you must break the chains of the circle using these three steps:

1. **Calm** the physical symptoms of anxiety. Live in the moment and use relaxation techniques.
2. **Challenge** your anxious thoughts and look for problematic thinking patterns.
3. **Discover and stop** the behaviors that maintain and worsen your anxiety, such as avoiding situations or criticizing yourself.

Truth You Can Trust In

God's perfect love casts out fear (see 1 John 4:18); His Word shows us truth that we can cling to when we experience anxiety and fear. Keep your mind focused on the truth in His Word.

- God gives us a spirit of power and self-control. Anxiety and fear are liars, tools of the enemy.
  FEAR: F – False **E** – Evidence **A** – Appearing **R** – Real

  For God gave us a spirit not of fear but of power and love and self-control. (2 Timothy 1:7)

- He will strengthen you to handle life's stressors.

  Fear not, for I am with you; be not dismayed, for I am your God; I will strengthen you, I will help you, I will uphold you with my righteous right hand. (Isaiah 41:10)

- He will supply your every need.

  And my God will supply every need of yours according to his riches in glory in Christ Jesus. (Philippians 4:19)

- He gives us a purpose and a future. We do not need to worry about the future.

  For I know the plans I have for you, declares the LORD, plans for welfare and not for evil, to give you a future and a hope. (Jeremiah 29:11)

  Even to your old age I am he, and to gray hairs I will carry you. I have made, and I will bear; I will carry and will save. (Isaiah 46:4)

- You can move on!

  I press on toward the goal for the prize of the upward call of God in Christ Jesus. (Philippians 3:14)

Strategy: R.E.A.S.O.N.

*Trade in the chaos of anxiety for reason! We will have stressors in life. James 1:2 says to "Count it all joy, my brothers, when you meet trials of various kinds," but the one suffering with anxiety feels a need to control the trials instead of rejoicing in them. Learning to deal with anxiety in a healthy, biblical way **allows anxiety to work for you instead of controlling you**. Remember the acrostic R.E.A.S.O.N. for dealing with anxiety:*

Relax

Relax your body and slow your breathing. Anxiety clouds your mind, preparing your body to fight or flee. This causes an adrenalin rush, rapid heartbeat, muscle tension, etc. Your body is not preparing your mind to think, but to take emergency action. By calming your physical response, you can clear your mind. (See the end of this chapter for relaxation tools.)

Examine

Examine your surroundings to help ground you in the moment. Stay in the here and now. Focus on an object in your hand, or do a task like washing dishes, and focus only on that task.

> *Therefore do not be anxious about tomorrow, for tomorrow will be anxious for itself. Sufficient for the day is its own trouble. (Matthew 6:34)*

Actual

Is there an actual threat or a real reason for your anxiety? Search your surroundings. Is there an external threat? What are the triggers?

Shift

Shift your mindset. Peace comes when your mind is stayed on the Lord. Meditate on the Word of the Lord and His truths; do not allow what you feel or see to deceive you.

> *You keep him in perfect peace whose mind is stayed on you, because he trusts in you. (Isaiah 26:3)*

> *Finally, brothers, whatever is true, whatever is honorable, whatever is just, whatever is pure, whatever is lovely, whatever is commendable, if there is any excellence, if there is anything worthy of praise, think about these things. (Philippians 4:8)*

Offer

Offer your burden to the Lord. Pray with gratitude in your heart for all God has done. It is difficult to worry about the future when you reflect on how the Lord has helped and blessed you in the past. Humble yourself and do not look to your own wisdom or try to take control. Give your anxieties to God and give Him the responsibility for the outcome.

> *Do not be anxious about anything, but in everything by prayer and supplication with thanksgiving let your requests be made known to God. (Philippians 4:6)*

> *Humble yourselves, therefore, under the mighty hand of God so that at the proper time he may exalt you, casting all your anxieties on him, because he cares for you. (1 Peter 5:6 – 7)*

New Thinking

Renew your mind and think differently. Changing how you process information involves seeking truth and rejecting messages that reinforce insecurity, pain, shame, and fear from past situations. Seek wisdom to discern truth from the problematic thinking prompting your anxiety.

> *If any of you lacks wisdom, let him ask God, who gives generously to all without reproach, and it will be given him. (James 1:5)*

Calming and Relaxation

With anxiety, your clouded mind makes relaxation difficult. Employing simple techniques to help clear your mind and calm physical sensations will give you the ability to handle anxiety and panic. For people who experience anxiety daily, the body adapts to the nervous, jittery feelings, and this becomes the new normal for them. Over time, intentional relaxation can reduce the amount of tension the body considers "normal."

Be careful not to use relaxation techniques as an excuse not to deal with the underlying issues causing your anxiety. This is a danger of this technique. When you feel and function better, it is easier to fall into avoidance rather than to deal with what is making you uncomfortable.

You may be tempted to skip relaxation exercises unless you are experiencing extreme anxiety or panic, but this is also a mistake. **Using relaxation only to stop panic, rather than using it to prevent panic, sends a message to your brain that anxiety is bad.** Anxiety is a normal emotion that everyone experiences in response to a perceived threat. When your brain treats anxiety as the threat, any moment that would trigger normal anxiety creates a strong anxious response. Your mind is responding to dual threats: the trigger and the anxiety. **It is as if you become afraid to fear.**

Relax Safely

Use the following guidelines for relaxation as a **preemptive**, routine practice. Treat relaxation as exercise. The more you do it, the stronger you get at it. Make relaxation part of your daily routine. Be intentional. Set time aside to relax in the morning, and before and after stressful situations. This will help you cope with life instead of avoiding it. These transformational techniques are so simple that you can do them anywhere, and they only take a few minutes.

> ### Questions to Ponder
> Read the REASON strategy and put it into practice.
>
> **30.1) Write about using the strategy.**
>
> **30.2) How did the strategy help you?**
>
> **30.3) Where did you find the strategy difficult to implement?**
>
> **30.4) How do you relax? Write the ways you currently relax.**
>
> **30.5) How often do you spend time relaxing?**
>
> **30.6) What activities do you enjoy that your anxiety prevents you from doing?**
>
> **30.7) Try the relaxation techniques that follow. How do you feel about using these techniques?**

Slow your body down to help your mind get through difficult episodes of anxiety.

For God alone, O my soul, wait in silence, for my hope is from him. (Psalm 62:5)

Relaxation Techniques

Just Breathe — Rectangle

1. Breathe in from your diaphragm, not your chest. Fold your hands on your belly and notice your belly fill with air.

2. Do not take extra deep breaths. The point is to slow your breathing, not take in more air.

3. Picture a rectangle in your mind. Breathe in slowly to the count of five as you follow an imaginary rectangle in your mind.

4. Hold your breath to the count of three. Exhale slowly to the count of five and then hold to the count of three. Continue to follow the rectangle in your mind.

5. Repeat for about 10 minutes. Do this exercise each morning, evening, and when a situation overwhelms you, before the anxiety becomes severe.

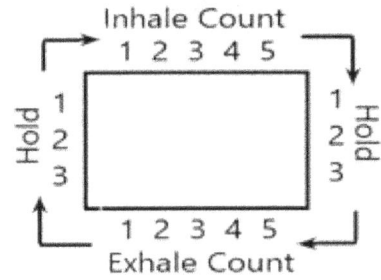

Inhale Count
1 2 3 4 5
Hold 1 2 3
Hold 1 2 3
1 2 3 4 5
Exhale Count

Slow Your Mind

Racing thoughts accompany anxiety. When your mind spins up, guided by unclear thoughts, it creates pressure to act. When your efforts to regain control of your mind fail, anxiety increases. Realize it is not possible to stop a thought from entering your mind. The problem is not your thought, but what you do with it. **A thought is just a thought.** It can be truth or a lie, but it cannot hurt you. **You need not act on the thought or control it.** When anxiety comes, observe your thoughts and let the anxiety pass through you and out of you like a wave; ride the wave to dry ground.

Ride the wave:

1. **Relax.** Tense and relax each muscle in your body one at a time until your entire body relaxes, notice the thoughts and sensations of anxiety flowing through and out of you like a wave.

2. **Do you feel safe?** God is your safe place. Secure yourself in the Lord. When you know you are in a safe place, you can observe your thoughts without interacting with them.

3. **Self-talk.** Remind yourself that nothing is going to hurt you and that this wave will end. If you can identify a specific thought, take it captive and focus on how the Lord's truth applies to it.

4. **Redirect your thoughts.** Do an activity or focus on something tangible. For example, hold a cold glass in your hand, focusing on the temperature of the glass, the texture, the size. Concentrate on the solid ground underneath each step you take. Do a chore like dishes, focusing on the water texture, the cloth, the motion of the towel, and so on.

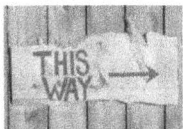

> Self-care is vital to recovery from anxiety. This includes good sleep, good diet, exercise, setting goals, relating well with others, and doing activities you enjoy. If anxiety interferes with your ability to live a productive life, **ask your coach for additional resources.**

Lesson 31 — A Completed Inventory

A New "Heart Check Plan"

Progress Check and New Goals

You have completed the inventory of your past and examined patterns in your thoughts and actions. You may see how one event from your life set the stage for other events. Most likely, this information has changed how you think about your life, yourself, and God, and influenced a different way of dealing with situations.

Look at the "Heart Check Plan" that you created before starting your inventory. What progress have you made towards achieving your goals? Have your goals changed?

_____
_____
_____
_____
_____
_____

Make New Goals or Write the Goals You Are Still Working Toward

List the areas you wish to correct	For each item you wish to correct, write the result you want to see.
_____	_____
_____	_____
_____	_____
_____	_____
_____	_____
_____	_____
_____	_____
_____	_____
_____	_____
_____	_____
_____	_____
_____	_____
_____	_____
_____	_____
_____	_____

Visit the website at:

www.rebuiltrecovery.org

for downloadable pages and
more helpful resources!

www.ingramcontent.com/pod-product-compliance
Lightning Source LLC
Chambersburg PA
CBHW080423030426
42335CB00020B/2563